INTERPRETING CARDIAC ELECTROGRAMS - FROM SKIN TO ENDOCARDIUM

Edited by **Kevin A. Michael**

Interpreting Cardiac Electrograms - From Skin to Endocardium
http://dx.doi.org/10.5772/65202
Edited by Kevin A. Michael

Contributors

Pedro-Eduardo Alvarado-Rubio, Ricardo Mansilla, Lizette Segura, Alejandro Gonzalez, Miguel A. Becerra, Andrés Orozco, Juan Pablo Ugarte, Catalina Tobón, Javier Sainz, Xin Gao, Ioana Mozos, Dana I Stoian, Erik Wissner, Sorin Lazar, Gabriel Cismaru, Madhur Dev Bhattarai, Fariha Sadiq Ali, Sanoj Chacko

Published by InTech
Janeza Trdine 9, 51000 Rijeka, Croatia

Publishing Process Manager Maja Bozicevic
Technical Editor SPi Global
Cover InTech Design team

First published October, 2017
Printed in Croatia
Legal deposit, Croatia: National and University Library in Zagreb

Additional hard copies can be obtained from orders@intechopen.com

Interpreting Cardiac Electrograms - From Skin to Endocardium, Edited by Kevin A. Michael
p. cm.
Print ISBN 978-953-51-3571-5
Online ISBN 978-953-51-3572-2

For EU product safety concerns:
IN TECH d.o.o., Prolaz Marije Krucifikse Kozulić 3, 51000 Rijeka, Croatia,
info@intechopen.com or visit our website at intechopen.com.

Meet the editor

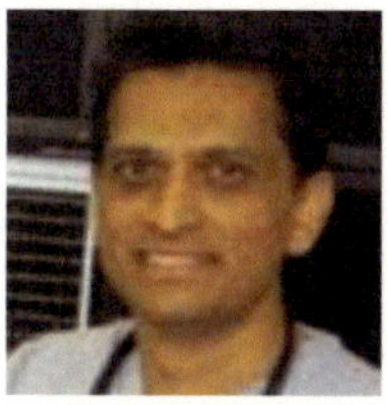

Kevin A. Michael graduated from the University of Natal in South Africa with a bachelor's degree in Medicine and Surgery (MBChB), and a master's degree in Cardiology (MPhil) from the University of Cape Town. He trained in internal medicine and cardiology at King Edward VIII Hospital and Groote Schuur Hospital in Cape Town, respectively. He was admitted as a fellow of the College of Physicians of South Africa in 2001 and was awarded his Certification in Cardiology through the Colleges of Medicine of South Africa in 2004. He completed a research fellowship at Southampton University Hospital in the United Kingdom and completed clinical fellowship training in cardiac electrophysiology at Queen's University in 2009. He was awarded his doctorate in Medicine from the University of Cape Town in 2013 based on his thesis examining defibrillation vectors and waveforms. Dr. Michael was appointed as assistant professor in the Department of Medicine at Queen's University, Ontario, Canada, and thereafter was promoted to Associate Professor attached to the Heart Rhythm Service, Kingston Health Sciences Unit in Ontario. He also serves as a consultant electrophysiologist at the Heart Rhythm Management Centre at Life Westville Hospital in Durban, South Africa. He retains an interest in complex ablation and cardiac defibrillation and pursues research both in a basic science and in a clinical capacity.

Contents

Preface

Firstly, I want to thank each of the authors for their contributions to this interesting and unique book project.

It certainly represents a tour de force and expansive review of cardiac electrogram interpretation intended for the advanced reader but highlighting certain basic concepts as well. These individual sections represent both works that are directly derived from clinical studies and relevant anecdotal cases as well as chapters on clinically relevant basic science.

Individual manuscripts have been compiled and edited to constitute the chapters. Each chapter tries to maintain the focus on interpreting the studies and data in a clinically relevant format that can be translated to patient care. The latter chapters in this body of work focus on the potential of innovative electrograms that have been mathematically derived and correlated to patient outcomes.

The first section examines the surface ECG. This is by no means a basic review of an approach to ECG readings but rather assumes that the reader is at an advanced level and starts off by introducing a diagnostic algorithm that Dr. Chacko et al. propose for diagnosing supraventricular tachycardias.

Left axis deviation on the ECG is explored by Dr. Madhur.

I am pleased to also include a chapter that addresses the diagnostic potential of the signal-averaged ECG.

This highly useful surface of electrogram derivation has certainly been neglected by general physicians as well as cardiologists alike and is a useful way of amplifying low amplitude cardiac potentials that can explain the mechanism or assess the potential risk of ventricular arrhythmias. This manuscript by Ioana et al. starts by reinforcing the diagnostic criteria of the signal-averaged ECG and thereafter explores its application.

The contribution by Dr. Xin Gao looks specifically at the fetal ECG and the filtering required in order to discern more clearly fetal heart rate monitoring. This potential may lead to the detection of fetal arrhythmias in utero.

In the second section of this book, manuscripts that interpret electrograms from intracardiac pacemakers and implantable cardioverter-defibrillators (ICDs) are examined in closer detail.

Both Dr. Erik Wissner et al. and Dr. Sadiq Ali et al. look at the interpretation of these device electrograms for the purposes of diagnosis and troubleshooting of ICDs, and Dr. Cismaru Gabriel et al. specifically examine the intracardiac electrograms from ICDs implanted in patients with Brugada syndrome. This section is not only relevant for the elimination of inappropriate therapies, which still plague patients with ICDs and various studies quote incidences of up to 16%, but also addresses the concept of a more standardized programming for both primary and secondary indications.

The concept of mere "shock box" single-zone programming for primary prevention is challenged and summarized by examining all recent randomized controlled trials. The strategy proposed is to employ multiple VT detection zones and apply advanced detection algorithms in all zones given the advancement and high specificity of these algorithms, which include morphological discriminators in most devices.

The section on the Brugada syndrome examines specifically the morphological interpretation of the specific intracardiac signals during ventricular arrhythmias in this disease.

This is brought to clinical relevance by proposing to use the stored ICD events and electrograms (EGMs) to plan and guide mapping and catheter ablation both in the case of monomorphic re-entry ventricular tachycardia and in the case of Brugada syndrome, ablation of PVC triggers that initiate VF. Each of these concepts is well illustrated with case studies and actual patient intracardiac electrograms (EGMs).

The final section in this book looks at various basic science concepts in a clinically applied context. Catalina Tobón et al. review complex fractionation from intracardiac EGM sources using nonlinear signal analysis. The concept of targeting complex fractionated electrograms (CFE) during ablation for persistent and long-standing persistent atrial fibrillation (AF) has been controversial. More recently, ablation of cardiac ganglia, specific optical mapping and ablation AF rotors have entered the arena. Various studies have been proposed that examine atrial fibrillation CFE signals in order to see if they exhibit temporospatial stability and if these signals can be used as a surrogate marker to identify rotors.

The final manuscript in this book proposes a controversial concept of using a bioelectrical signal derived from surface electrocardiograms in patients to predict the prognosis in patients. It is not a replacement for the 12 lead ECGs but is an interesting additional concept that has been explored in other studies. The data are at best anecdotal and need refinement, but nevertheless warrant closer scrutiny.

In summary, this book as a collation of manuscripts incorporates clinical data and basic science concepts in relation to cardiac signal processing and interpretation.

Kevin A. Michael, MBChB, MPhil, MD
Associate Professor, Department of Medicine, Queen's University
Kingston, Ontario, Canada

Section 1

Concepts from the Surface Electrocardiogram

Chapter 1

An Approach to Diagnosing Supraventricular Tachycardias on the 12-Lead ECG

Sanoj Chacko and Adrian Baranchuk

Additional information is available at the end of the chapter

http://dx.doi.org/10.5772/intechopen.70143

Abstract

Supraventricular tachycardia (SVT) is a general term describing a group of arrhythmias whose mechanism involves the atria and atrioventricular nodal tissue for its initiation and maintenance. SVT is a common entity in clinical practice with a prevalence of 2.25 cases per 1000 in general population. Atrial fibrillation and atrial flutter are the most common presentations of SVTs. Of the remaining subtypes of SVT, atrioventricular nodal re-entrant tachycardia (AVNRT) accounts for 60% of the cases. The atrioventricular re-entrant tachycardia (AVRT) and atrial tachycardia (AT) represent approximately 30 and 10% of the cases, respectively. The mechanisms of different forms of SVT have been elucidated and are caused by either re-entrant circuit, increased automaticity or triggered activity. This chapter provides an overview of how to systematically approach a narrow complex tachycardia.

Keywords: supraventricular tachycardia, atrioventricular nodal re-entry tachycardia, atrioventricular re-entry tachycardia, atrial tachycardia, atrial fibrillation, atrial flutter

1. Introduction

A systematic approach in the interpretation of ECG is important to arrive at a definitive diagnosis of the subtype of supraventricular tachycardia (SVT). Narrow complex tachycardias (NCT) are broadly divided as regular or irregular tachycardia. Irregular NCT are either atrial fibrillation or atrial flutter with variable ventricular response. For a regular NCT, the next key step would be to identify the presence of a P wave, positive or negative P waves, and its morphology and location of the P wave with respect to the cardiac cycle. Absence of P wave in a regular NCT narrows the differential diagnosis to either typical atrioventricular nodal re-entrant tachycardia (AVNRT) or junctional tachycardia. If the P waves are positive and are located before the QRS complex, it is likely to be sinus tachycardia. On the other hand, if the P waves are negative, that excludes a sinus origin of the rhythm. A negative P wave in front of the QRS complex implies a low atrial tachycardia (LAT). If the P waves embedded in the QRS complex have a short RP interval, it is described as short RP tachycardia, and the differentials would include typical AVNRT or atrioventricular re-entrant tachycardia (AVRT). If the RP interval is longer than the PR interval, the tachycardia is termed as long RP tachycardia, and the differentials would include atypical AVNRT or atrial tachycardia (AT) [1, 2]. The algorithm in **Figure 1** shows the flow chart of how to systematically approach a NCT.

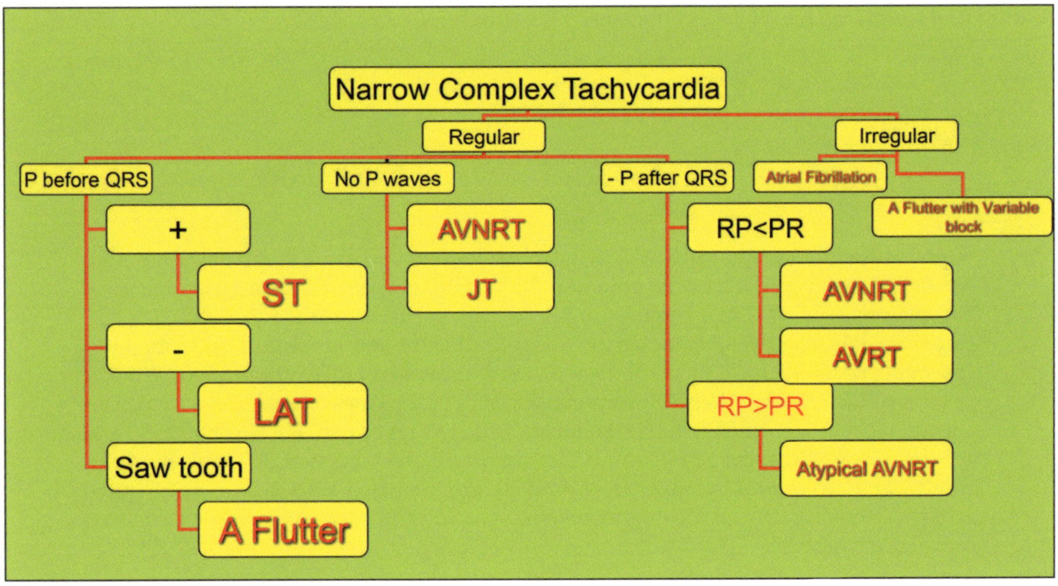

Figure 1. Algorithm for narrow complex tachycardia.

2. Subtypes of NCTs

1. Sinus tachycardia
2. Atrial fibrillation
3. Atrial flutter
4. Low atrial tachycardia
5. Typical AVNRT
6. Atypical AVNRT
7. Orthodromic AVRT
8. Junctional tachycardia

2.1. Sinus tachycardia

Sinus tachycardia is a normal physiological response to exercise or pathology in which catecholamine release is enhanced. Sinus tachycardia is described as inappropriate sinus tachycardia (IST), when individuals present with chronic non-paroxysmal sinus tachycardia, with a structurally normal heart and with no apparent causes for sinus tachycardia. Sinus tachycardia is also noted in young individuals with structurally normal heart, in whom there is an exaggerated heart rate response to upright position, termed as postural orthostatic tachycardia syndrome (POTS). ECG in **Figure 2** is an example of a regular narrow complex tachycardia with upright P-waves in front of QRS complex, in leads I and II indicating a sinus origin with 1:1 relationship, consistent with sinus tachycardia. Vagal maneuvers or atrioventricular (AV) nodal blocking agents may be useful in further determining the mechanism of tachycardia. **Figure 3** is an ECG of a patient with cardiac tamponade, showing sinus tachycardia with electrical alternans.

2.2. Atrial tachycardia (AT)

AT is a regular atrial rhythm originating from an ectopic focus either from the right or left atrium. Focal AT is usually paroxysmal but can also present as incessant tachycardia, causing left ventricular systolic dysfunction. Right ATs are usually located in the tricuspid annulus followed by crista terminalis, coronary sinus ostium, and perinodal tissues in the order of frequency. Similarly, the left ATs predominantly originate from the pulmonary veins followed by mitral annulus, interatrial septum, and left atrial appendage. Classically, an ECG reveals negative P waves in the inferior leads, suggesting a caudo-cranial atrial activation (**Figure 4**).

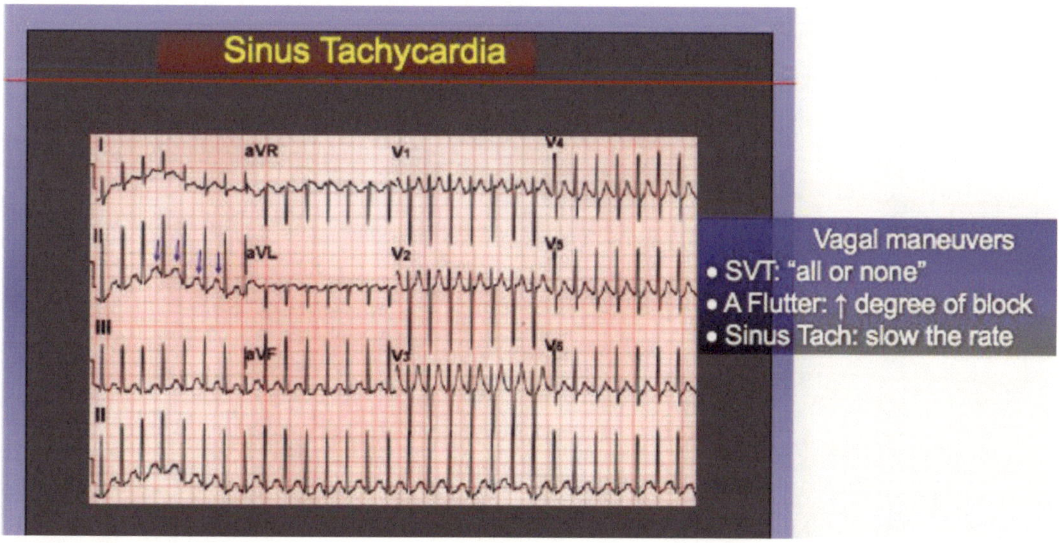

Figure 2. ECG showing sinus tachycardia with upright P-wave before the QRS complex (blue arrow) indicating sinus origin with 1:1 AV relationship.

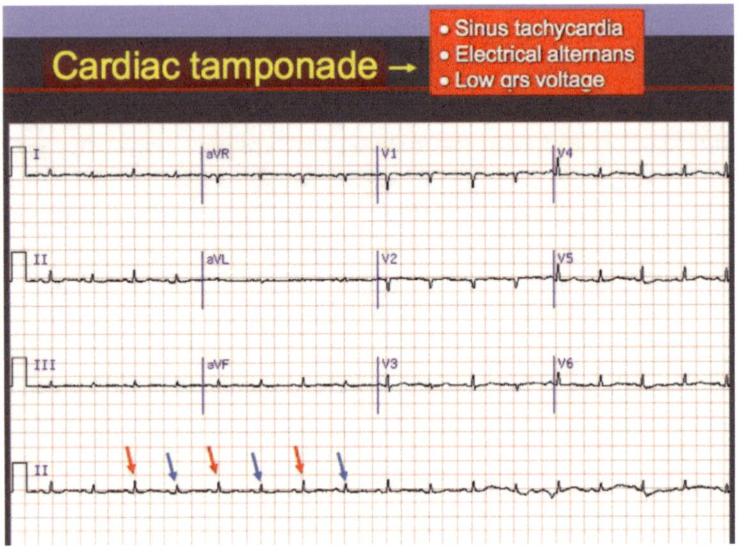

Figure 3. ECG showing sinus tachycardia with low QRS voltage and electrical alternans in a patient with cardiac tamponade.

2.3. Atrioventricular nodal re-entrant tachycardia (AVNRT)

Patients with AVNRT demonstrate dual AV nodal physiology, fast pathway with long refractory period and slow pathway with short refractory period. While 25–30% of the general population

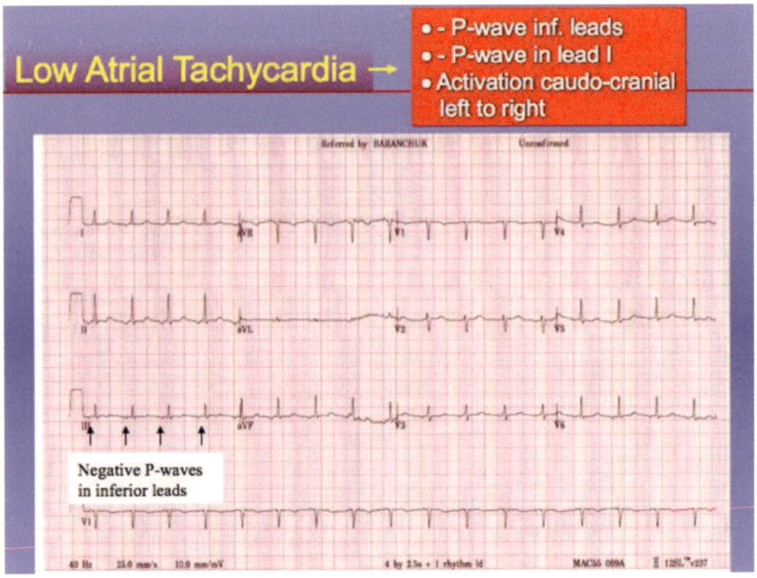

Figure 4. ECG showing negative P-waves in the inferior leads and lead I with caudo-cranial activation consistent with low atrial tachycardia.

has dual AV nodal physiology, only a minority of them develop AVNRT. Typically, a critically timed premature atrial contraction (PAC) initiates the tachycardia and the classical symptom involves abrupt onset and offset of palpitations. Typical AVNRT accounts for 80–90% of all AVNRTs. In slow–fast AVNRT, the antegrade conduction occurs through the slow pathway and retrograde conduction through the fast pathway. The 12-lead ECG typically shows a narrow complex tachycardia with absent P waves or retrograde P waves and RP interval of <100 ms (**Figure 5**) [3]. In atypical AVNRT, the antegrade conduction occurs down the fast pathway and retrograde conduction up the slow pathway [4], and the 12-lead ECG will reveal a narrow complex tachycardia, with RP > PR interval, termed as long RP tachycardia.

2.4. Atrioventricular re-entrant tachycardia (AVRT)

AVRT is a re-entrant tachycardia with a circuit that consists of two distinct pathways, normal AV nodal conduction system and the accessory pathway. The accessory pathway may manifest as preexcitation in the surface ECG (delta wave) if the antegrade conduction is exclusively through the pathway or a combination of pathway and AV node or concealed (without preexcitation) if the conduction is exclusively through the AV node. AVRT is classified as orthodromic if the antegrade conduction occurs via the AV node and antidromic if antegrade conduction occurs through the accessory pathway. Orthodromic AVRT accounts for 90–95% of the AVRTs associated with Wolf-Parkinson-White (WPW) syndrome [5]. **Figure 6** shows a routine surface ECG of a young patient performed prior to a dental extraction. An ECG reveals preexcitation with positive delta wave in inferior leads, I, aVL, and negative delta

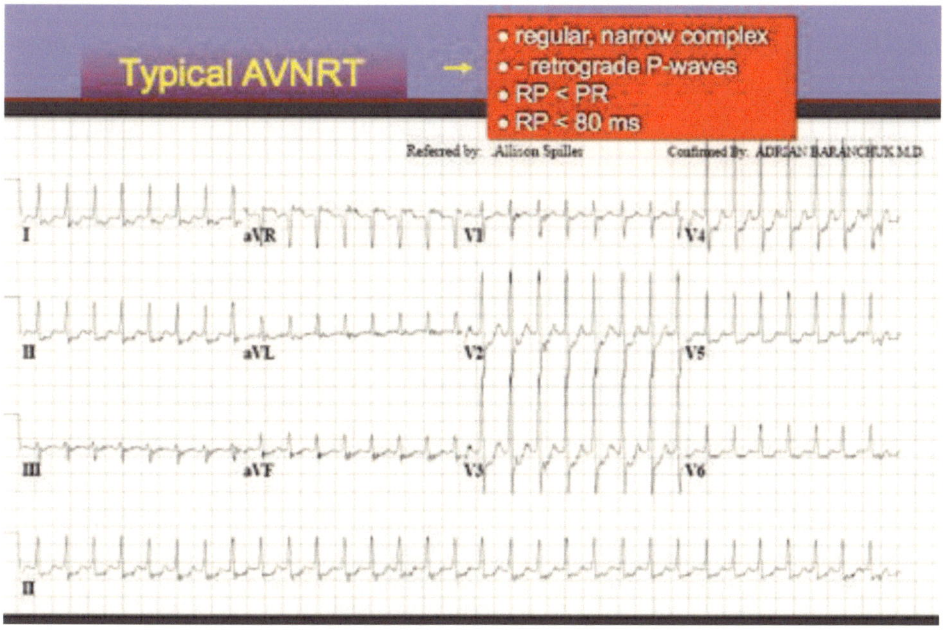

Figure 5. ECG showing regular narrow complex tachycardia with retrograde P waves. Short RP (RP < PR) tachycardia with a RP interval of <100 ms.

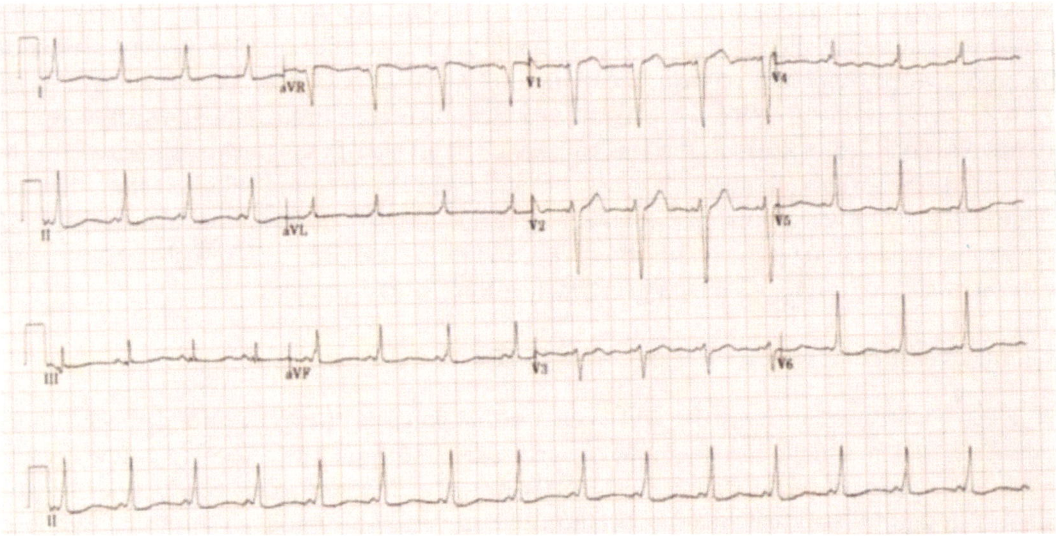

Figure 6. Surface ECG showing preexcitation with positive delta wave in inferior leads and I, aVL and negative delta wave in V1 consistent with a right anteroseptal accessory pathway.

wave in V1 consistent with possible right anteroseptal accessory pathway. **Figures 7** and **8** show a narrow complex tachycardia with retrograde P waves and long ventriculoatrial (VA) time consistent with orthodromic AVRT.

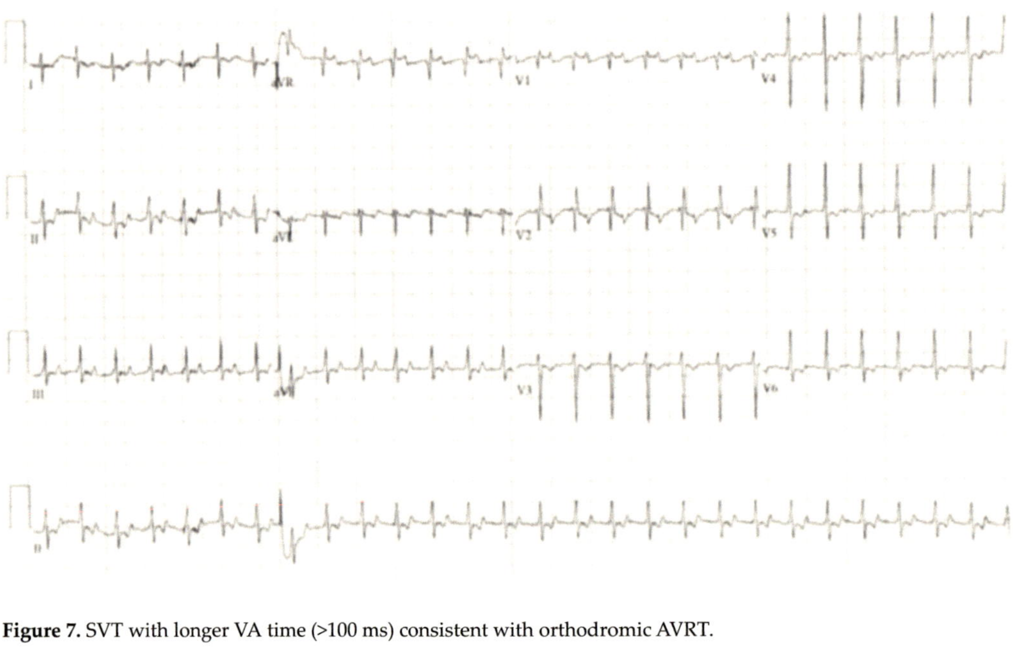

Figure 7. SVT with longer VA time (>100 ms) consistent with orthodromic AVRT.

http://dx.doi.org/10.5772/intechopen.70143

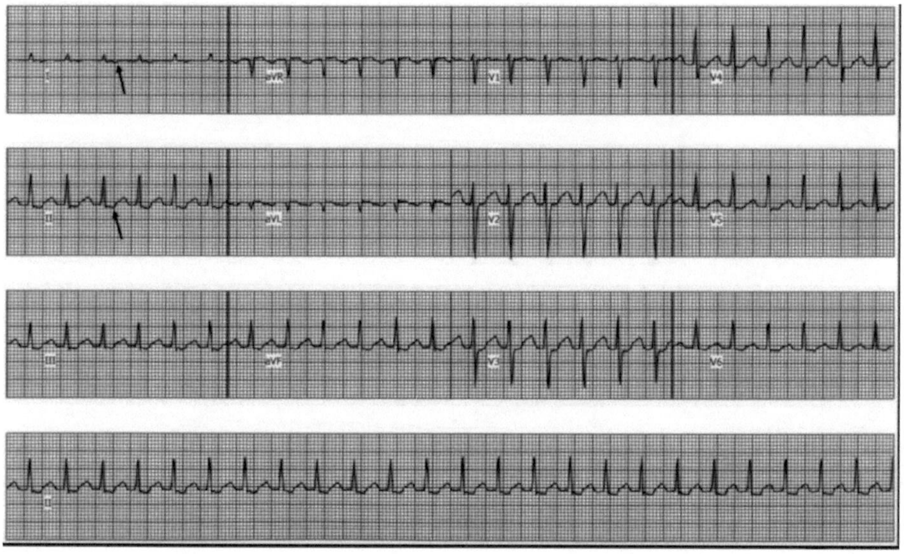

Figure 8. Regular narrow complex tachycardia with retrograde P-waves (black arrows), RP < PR and RP > 100 ms.

3. SVT with aberrancy

Narrow complex SVT may present as wide complex rhythm in the setting of aberrant conduction or the presence of accessory pathway. This can pose a diagnostic dilemma in differentiating from ventricular tachycardia (VT). Accurate differentiation of SVT-A from VT is challenging but is key to decision making and management in the emergency setting. In an effort to distinguish between VT and SVT with aberrancy, Brugada and Wellen proposed criteria to help determine the diagnosis [6].

Brugada and Wellen's criteria

1. Absence of RS complexes in all precordial leads
2. R to S interval >100 ms in one precordial lead
3. AV dissociation
4. Morphology criteria of VT in precordial leads
5. Precordial QRS concordance
6. Capture or fusion beats
7. Left axis deviation

An ECG in **Figure 9** is an example of SVT with aberrant conduction, on a patient who presented with palpitation. Rhythm strip shows regular P waves with 1:1 atrioventricular conduction. In addition, an ECG does not meet any of the above criteria for VT. An ECG in **Figure 10** shows a wide complex tachycardia with pseudo "RBBB" morphology, R to S >100 ms in the pseudo "LBBB" morphology leads, and 2:1 VA conduction, consistent with VT.

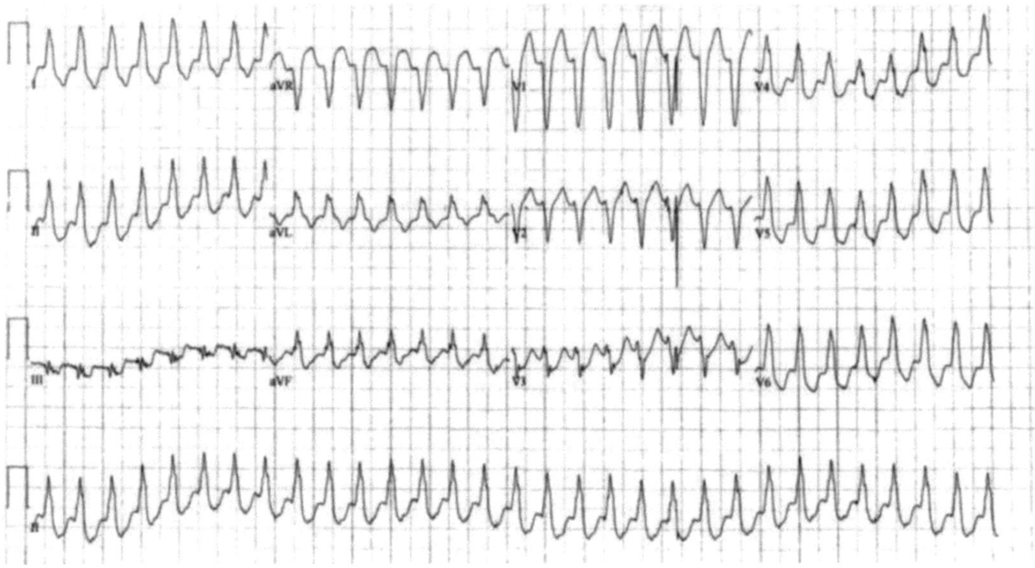

Figure 9. SVT with aberrancy.

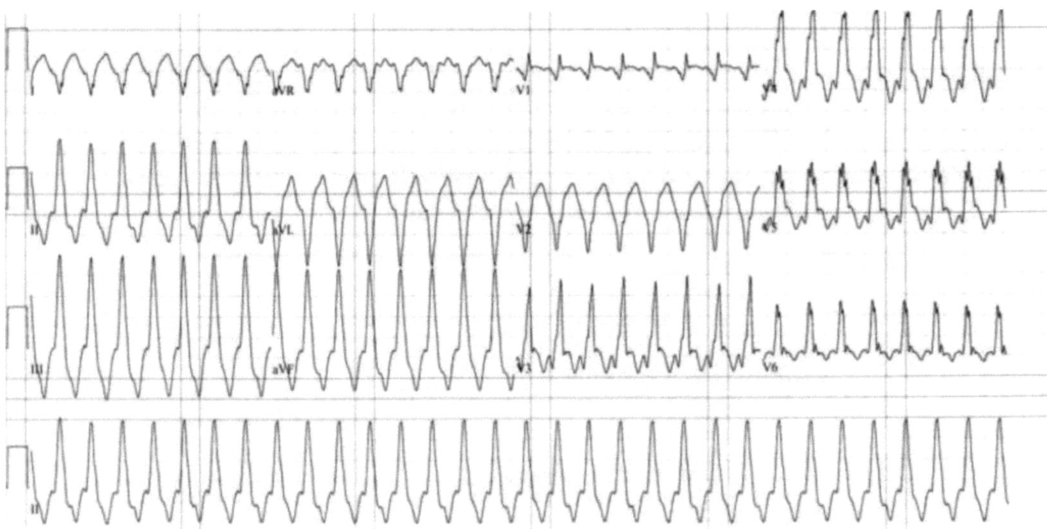

Figure 10. ECG showing wide complex tachycardia, RBBB morphology, R to S >100 ms in V2, and 2:1 VA (blue arrows) conduction consistent with VT.

4. Conclusion

SVT includes a variety of tachycardias originating from the atria and atrioventricular nodal tissues. The subtypes of SVT differ in their physiological mechanism and presentation. The unpredictability of the episodes and inability to control the disabling symptoms can render the patient incapacitated. Accurate diagnosis of the subtypes of SVT is essential to deliver the most appropriate therapy. Despite the highly specified symptomatic and ECG diagnostic criteria, arriving at a diagnosis is not always straightforward. A systematic approach to interpreting ECG is therefore crucial to narrow the differential diagnosis. Careful interpretation of ECGs can unfold important information, depict the underlying mechanism, and aid with the diagnosis and management.

Author details

Sanoj Chacko[1] and Adrian Baranchuk[2]*

*Address all correspondence to: barancha@kgh.kari.net

1 Heart Rhythm Service, Kingston General Hospital, Queen's University, Kingston, Ontario, Canada

2 Division of Cardiology, Department of Medicine, Kingston General Hospital, Queen's University, Kingston, Ontario, Canada

References

[1] Antzelevitch C, Burashnikov A. Overview of basic mechanisms of cardiac arrhythmia. Cardiac Electrophysiology Clinics. 2011 Mar 1;**3**(1):23-45

[2] Kistler PM, Roberts-Thomson KC, Haqqani HM, et al. P-wave morphology in focal atrial tachycardia: Development of an algorithm to predict the anatomic site of origin. Journal of the American College of Cardiology. 2006 Sep 5;**48**(5):1010-1017

[3] Katritsis DG, Camm AJ. Classification and differential diagnosis of atrioventricular nodal re-entrant tachycardia. Europace. 2006;**8**:29-36

[4] Katritsis DG, Camm AJ. Atrioventricular nodal reentrant tachycardia. Circulation. 2010 Aug 24;**122**(8):831-840

[5] Blomström-Lundqvist C, Scheinman MM, Aliot EM, et al. ACC/AHA/ESC guidelines for the management of patients with supraventricular arrhythmias—executive summary: A report of the American College of Cardiology/American Heart Association Task Force on Practice Guidelines and the European Society of Cardiology Committee for Practice Guidelines (writing committee to develop guidelines for the management of patients with supraventricular arrhythmias) developed in collaboration with NASPE-Heart Rhythm Society. Journal of the American College of Cardiology. 2003 Oct 15;**42**(8):1493-1531

[6] Brugada P, Brugada J, Mont L, et al. A new approach to the differential diagnosis of a regular tachycardia with a wide QRS complex. Circulation. 1991;**83**:1649

Chapter 2

Examining Left Axis Deviation

Madhur Dev Bhattarai

Additional information is available at the end of the chapter

http://dx.doi.org/10.5772/intechopen.69435

Abstract

Axis deviation indicates possible presence of various conditions. It also affects the QRS and T morphologies. The limits of axis deviations are as such arbitrary and the approximate degree of axis itself can be easily determined. Various conditions often shift the QRS axis without fulfilling the defined limits of deviations in the initial stage. The associations with various conditions may be missed if such partial shift of the axis is disregarded. Isolated left axis deviation is relatively common in the general population and left anterior fascicular conduction delay is the most common cause of such isolated leftward shift of axis. Vulnerability of left anterior fascicle to interruption makes it likely to be affected by both atherosclerosis and fibrodegeneration. Glucose intolerance may increase the risk of both atherosclerosis and fibrodegeneration. The association of glucose intolerance with leftward shift of axis has been increasingly noticed. Research studies to get further evidences are required; however, utilizing the already available evidences to protect the susceptible population is equally essential. Documenting the approximate degree itself of the axis is the bottom line to study the association with the levels of various possible risk factors like glycated hemoglobin.

Keywords: ECG axis, left axis deviation, left anterior fascicular block, glucose intolerance, diabetes, diabetes prevention, indigenous population, ageing, Bachmann's bundle, neuropathy, white matter hyperintensities

1. Introduction

The limits for mean frontal plane QRS axis deviations are considered variedly [1–11] and are necessarily arbitrary [5]. In this chapter, determination of left axis deviation and its effects on QRS-T morphology and its causes will be discussed. The left axis deviation and leftward shift of axis have been increasingly noticed in asymptomatic relatively younger adults with diabetes. Next in the chapter, the epidemiology, pathogenesis, correlation with other related factors, and implications of the possible association between glucose intolerance and left axis deviation will be discussed.

2. The conducting system of the heart

In the heart, apart from ordinary myocardium and supporting fibrous skeleton, there are small groups of specialized neuromuscular cells in the myocardium which initiate and conduct cardiac electrical impulse [9, 12]. **Figure 1** shows the different parts of the specialized cardiac conducting system from the sinus node to the atrioventricular (AV) node with three internodal tracts in-between and then from the AV node to the His-Purkinje system [9, 12]. The atria and the ventricles are separated by a ring of fibrous tissue, which does not conduct electrical impulse. Thus, the electrical activity from the atria can only spread to the ventricles through the atrioventricular node and the atrioventricular bundle. Atrioventricular bundle (Bundle of His) originates from atrioventricular node and divides at the upper end of the ventricular system into right and left bundle branch [12]. The right

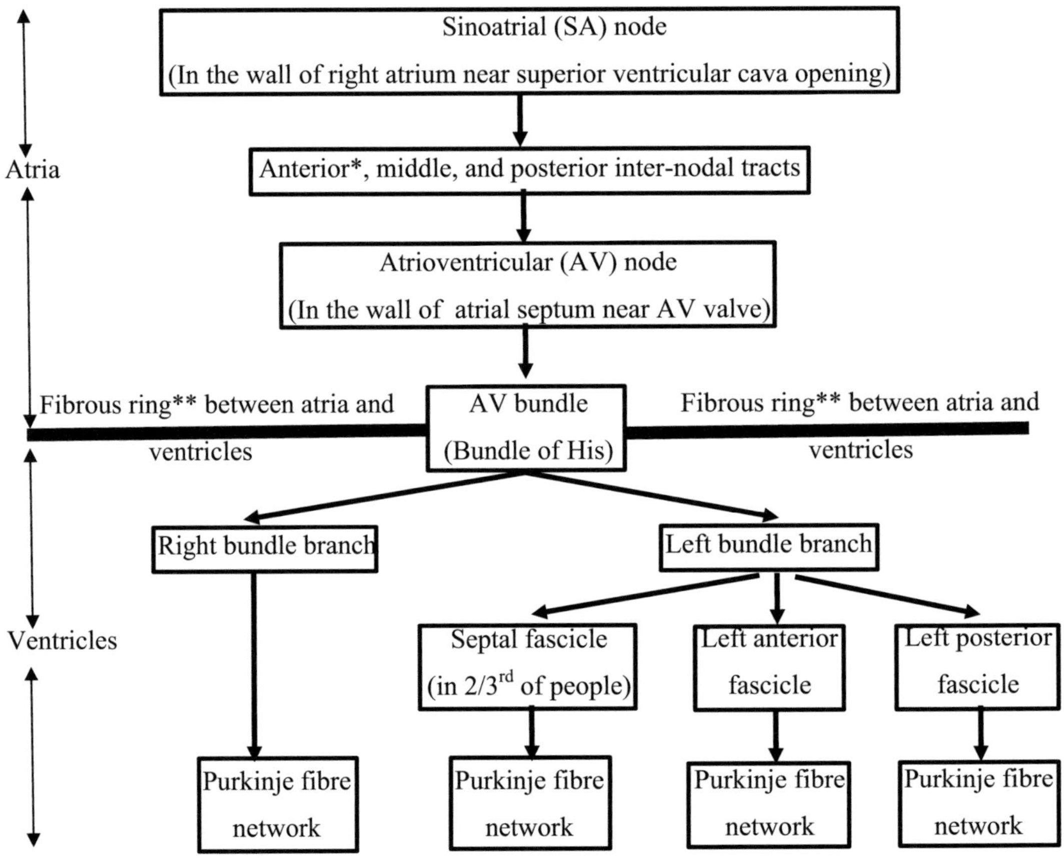

Figure 1. Different parts (shown in the boxes) of specialized cardiac conducting system from the sinoatrial node to the His-Purkinje system.
*Interatrial tract or the Bachmann's bundle is a branch of the anterior internodal tract to the left atrium which serves as the preferential path for electrical activation of the left atrium.
**Fibrous ring does not conduct electrical impulse.

bundle branch does not divide, but the left bundle branch further divides into three separate fascicles, namely septal (median or medial) fascicle, left anterior fascicle, and left posterior fascicle. Right bundle branch and different fascicles of left bundle branch ultimately break up within the ventricular myocardium into fine fibers as the network of Purkinje fibers [12]. The left anterior fascicular block (or the left anterior hemiblock) causes left axis deviation and the left posterior fascicular block (or left posterior hemiblock) causes right axis deviation. Isolated left posterior fascicular block is extremely rare [2, 5]. Septal fascicle is found in nearly two-thirds of people [13]. Delay or block of left septal fascicle may occur in diabetes, Chagas disease, and various cardiac diseases and may manifest in the ECG with prominent R waves in leads V1–V3, loss of septal Q waves, initial q waves in leads V1 and V2, and normal QRS axis [2]. However, the term left septal fascicular block is not recommended because of the lack of universally accepted criteria [3].

3. The normal mean frontal plane QRS axis range

An electrocardiogram is a record of the origin and propagation of the electric action potential through heart muscle. Depolarization spreads throughout the heart to stimulate the myocardium to contract and the vector demonstrates the direction in which depolarization is moving. The general, mean, or dominant direction of all these vectors is known as the mean vector and is expressed electrocardiographically as the mean QRS axis [2] which is located by degrees [1]. The direction of the mean QRS axis on the frontal plane is known as the mean frontal plane QRS axis and is determined by the six frontal plane limb leads; they are three standard bipolar limb leads I, II, and III and three augmented unipolar limb leads aVR, aVL, and aVF. The frontal plane limb leads are conventionally represented on a hexaxial reference system (**Figure 2**).

In most normal adults, the mean QRS vector points downward and to the left [1] with the electric axis of the QRS complex almost parallel to the anatomic base-to-apex axis of the heart in the direction of the lead II [6]. Most normal frontal plane QRS axes in the adults are directed within a narrower range between +40° and +60° [2], around 5 o'clock position [7] (**Figure 2**). Such range has been reported particularly at sea level from studies of axes conducted at different altitudes [14, 15]. Leads I and aVF, II and aVL, and III and aVR are at right angles to each other; that is, each of the pair is the right-angled partner leads. The concept of the right-angled partner leads (**Figure 2**) is helpful to quickly find the lead with the relatively tall R wave after looking at the lead with the equiphasic QRS complex. Coincidentally, but useful for remembering easily the pairs of the right-angled partner leads, the letters F, L, and R of the augmented limb leads are in the increasing alphabetic order like the numbers I, II, and III of the bipolar limb leads.

There are variations not only in the conventionally considered limits of normal axis and left, right, and extreme axis deviations in the adults but also in the nomenclature of the deviations and in the use of positive and negative signs of the degrees of the axis. The indicated limits of normal axis and left, right, and extreme axis deviations in the adults by various publications are shown below; for example

- **Normal axis** as 0° to +90° [1, 2], –30° to +90° [4, 6, 7, 10], and –30° to +100° [5, 9, 16].
- **Left axis deviation** as 0° to –90° [1, 2] and –30° to –90° [4–6, 10] with axis between 0° and –30° as *slight left axis deviation* [2], and between –30° and –45° as *moderate*, and between –45° and –90° as *marked left axis deviations* [3].
- **Right axis deviation** as +90° to 180° [2–4, 6], +90° to +150° [11], +100° to 180° [5, 16], +110° to 180° [9], +90° to –150° [10], and +90° to –90° [7].
- **Extreme axis deviation** as –90° to 180° [1, 2, 4–6] and –90° to –149° [10].

The extreme axis deviation [4–6] has also been

- included under right axis deviation [7],
- called as the northwest region axis [2], extreme right axis deviation [1], and extreme left axis deviation [9], and
- even indicated as the marked left or right axis deviation [5].

Similarly, there are variations in the use of + and – signs. For 180°,

- many use ± [2, 6, 9],
- some use both +180° and –180° in their axis range figure [7],
- others use + sign [5], and
- still others use no + or – sign to 180° [4, 16].

For other positive axis degrees many use + signs [2, 5–7, 9, 16] and some do not use + sign [3, 4].

In this chapter, *+ sign has been used for positive degree and – sign for negative degree*. As 0° and 180° are common to both positive and negative degree sides and there is no other similar degree to cause confusion, *no sign has been indicated for 0° and 180°*.

The consensus in these issues will help the communication among clinicians and between students and teachers especially during the examination of the student. However, even the consensually defined limits of normal axis and left, right, and extreme axis deviations should not make the clinicians and researchers to disregard the leftward or rightward shift of the axis from its usual range of degree (between +40° and +60°) in the adults (**Figure 2**). Otherwise the important correlation of the shift of axis with the patients' clinical condition or with the various factors in the research study may be missed; this is also further discussed later. With the possibility of easy determination of the approximate degree of axis by any clinicians and researches (see Section 4) and with the support of the computer interpretation of ECG readings at hand, the approximate degrees of the axis should be recorded.

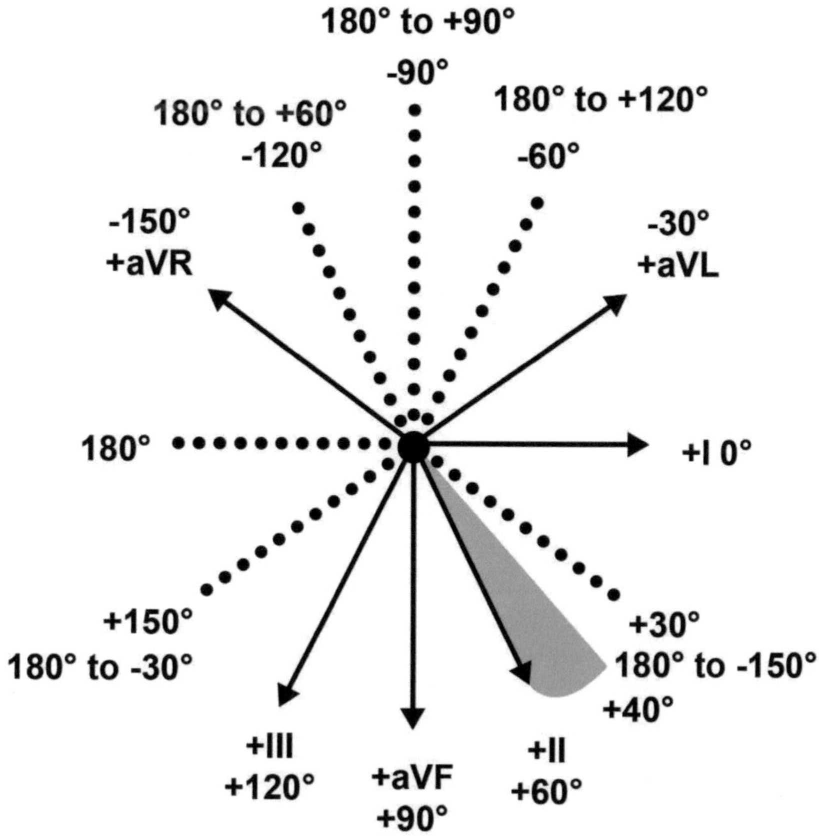

Figure 2. The frontal plane limb leads conventionally represented on a hexaxial reference system showing the range of degrees (between +40° and +60°) of most normal frontal QRS axes in the adults (shown as the shaded area). Note: **The positive and negative poles of each lead:** The arrow head on the solid line designates the positive pole of the corresponding lead axis and the dotted line the negative pole. **The 30° differences:** There are 30° differences between the positive or negative poles of the nearby leads. **The right-angled partner leads:** Leads I and aVF, II, and aVL, and III and aVR are at right angles to each other and the axis causing equiphasic deflections of QRS complex in one lead will cause maximum upward and downward deflections in the opposite ends of the other partner lead at right angle.

4. Determination of frontal plane QRS axis

4.1. Method of determining the approximate degree of mean axis

When depolarization moves in a direction with the cardiac axis toward the positive pole of a lead, the deflection recorded by the lead is upward (positive), if it is away from the positive pole it is negative (downward) and if it is perpendicular to the orientation of a lead the deflection recorded by the lead is isoelectric or equiphasic (QR or RS) QRS with equal magnitudes of upward (positive) and negative (downward) deflection [5]. The leads between the one recording the equiphasic (QR or RS) deflection and the other recording the maximum upward deflection will record the increasing degree of upward deflection; this area can be designated as *"positive-half area of the mean axis"* (**Figure 3**). Similarly, the leads

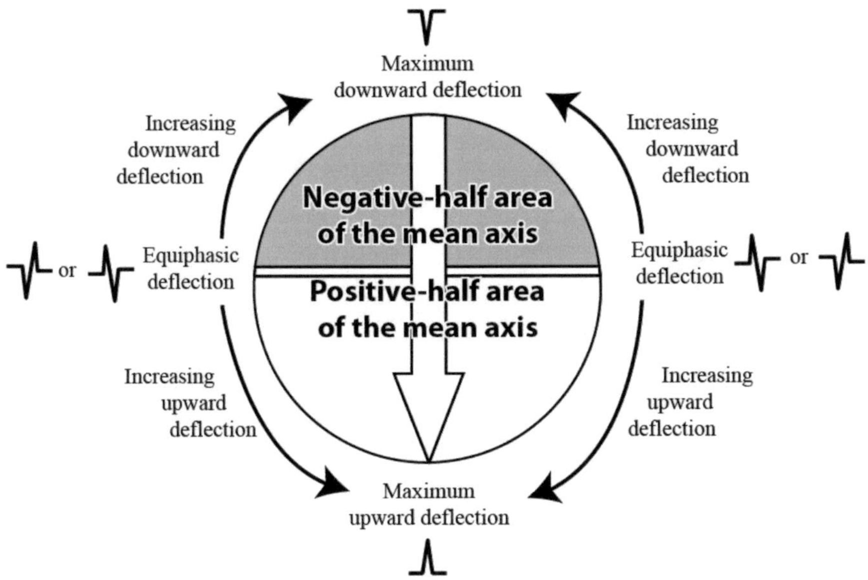

Figure 3. Varying degrees of upward or downward deflections recorded by different leads at various places in relation to the direction of cardiac axis (shown as the big central arrow). The leads in the "*positive-half area of the mean axis*" and "*negative-half area of the mean axis*" will record predominantly positive and negative QRS complex, respectively, increasingly so as per the distance from the points of equiphasic deflection (QR or RS).

between the one recording the equiphasic (QR or RS) deflection and the other recording the maximum downward deflection will record the increasing degree of downward deflection; this area can be designated as "*negative-half area of the mean axis.*" The mean QRS axis can, thus, be determined on the basis of one or both of the two rules [5]. As a general rule the mean QRS points

- midway between the axes of two extremity leads that show tall R waves of equal amplitude, and
- at 90° (right angle) to any extremity lead that shows a biphasic (QR or RS) complex and in the direction of leads that show relatively tall R waves [5].

With these considerations, the mean frontal plane QRS axis can be determined with an error of 10–15° [5]. Thus, to determine the approximate degree of axis, one has to find the lead in which the QRS complex is most equiphasic (QR or RS); the axis is directed perpendicular to this lead (**Figure 4**). If the lead with clear equiphasic QRS complex is not seen, then the lead having the QRS with the largest positive amplitude should be looked for. If there are two nearby leads which have almost equal tall R wave, the axis is mostly directed in between them (**Figure 4**).

The degree of the mean axis can be further reconfirmed by considering whether it is in accord or not with the QRS direction and amplitude in other leads in the areas in front of the line of the equiphasic complex, that is, in the *positive-half area of the mean axis* (**Figure 3**), and/or behind the line of the equiphasic complex, that is, in the *negative-half area of the mean axis*. This

http://dx.doi.org/10.5772/intechopen.69435

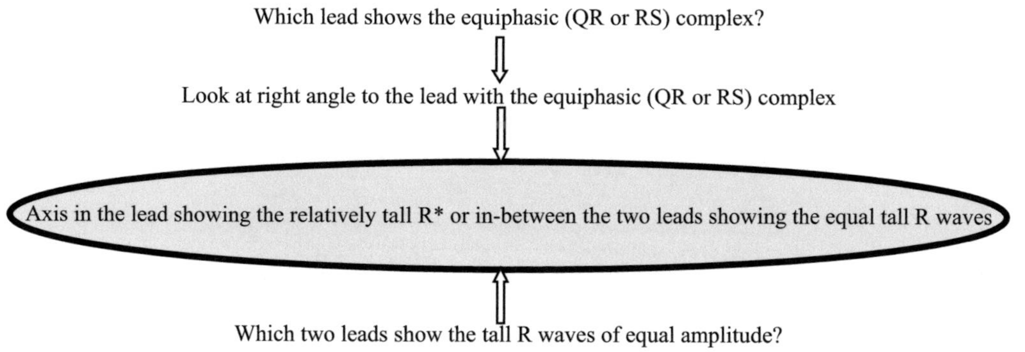

Figure 4. Method of determination of the approximate degree of the frontal plane QRS axis—The degree of the mean axis can be further reconfirmed by considering whether it is in accord or not with the QRS direction and amplitude in other leads in the areas in front of and/or behind the line of the equiphasic complex. *For example, if the relatively tall R wave is in the lead aVL the axis is approximately –30°, if in I it is 0°, if in II it is +60°, if in aVF it is +90°, if in III it is +120°, and if in aVR it is –150°.

method is perhaps the most appropriate observational technique to follow in the routine setting. The other method of the mean axis determination by plotting the net height or depth of two standard bipolar (not the augmented) limb leads [8, 9] is generally not practiced.

Sometimes an electrocardiogram with indeterminate QRS axis is encountered. In indeterminate QRS axis, the algebraic sum of major positive and major negative QRS waves is zero in each of leads I, II, and III, or the information from these three leads is incongruous [10]. In the absence of a dominant QRS deflection, as in an equiphasic QRS complex, the axis is said to be indeterminate [9]. The separate determination of the axes of the initial and later part of QRS complex may indicate, or help to correlate with, other findings. For example, in right bundle branch block (RBBB) the axis determination is of importance in diagnosing associated left anterior or posterior fascicular block, as right bundle branch on its own will not cause axis deviation. In right bundle branch block, estimating the frontal plane QRS based on the first 80–100 ms of the QRS deflection, primarily reflecting activation of the left ventricle, may help [4]. For left bundle branch block (LBBB) and other intraventricular delays, the entire QRS or just the initial 80–100 ms can be used [4].

4.2. An example of determination of the mean axis

An ECG with the recordings of the limb leads in an asymptomatic person is shown in **Figure 5** with left axis deviation. The QRS complex in II (which is at +60° in the hexaxial reference system) is most equiphasic; thus, the axis will be 90° to it, either in –30° or +150° (**Figure 2**). Since R wave in the lead aVL is positive and has almost the largest R wave amplitude, it dictates the direction of the vector. Thus, the QRS axis is leftward between around –30°. However, if we look carefully the lead II is not exactly equiphasic but it has slightly more negative complex especially the second QRS complex, so the lead II lies in the "*negative-half area of the mean axis*" (**Figure 3**). Similarly, the lead aVR is also near equiphasic with slightly more negative QRS complex, that is, the lead aVR is also in the "*negative-half area of the mean axis*" (**Figure 3**). As the

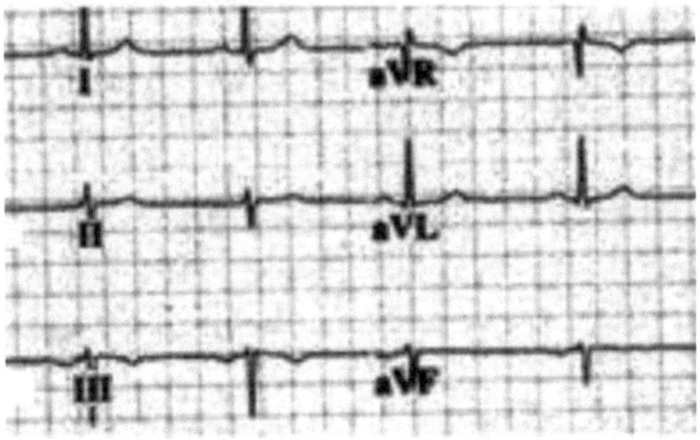

Figure 5. An electrocardiogram recording of the limb leads in an asymptomatic person.

lead II has slightly less negative QRS complex than the lead aVR, the lead II is slightly nearer to the mean axis than the aVR. So the mean axis is most likely around –40°.

In this example, we have determined the mean axis by first looking at the lead with the equiphasic QRS complex as described in **Figure 4** and later also reconfirm the degree of the mean axis by considering whether the QRS direction and amplitude in the leads in the *negative-half area* of the mean axis are in accord or not with it. As discussed above, the approximate determination of the axis with such method entails an error of 10–15° [5]. Moreover, minor degrees of change in the height of QRS complex may also occur due to the difference in the relative voltage and magnitude of the bipolar and augmented unipolar leads [9] or due to cardiac or respiratory movement.

4.3. Other axes

When cardiac axis is referred, it usually indicates the mean frontal plane QRS axis. But there are also other axes to consider, for example, T wave and P wave axes. Though even axis of ST segment [2] and the QRS axis in the horizontal plane [1, 6, 9] are also discussed, such axes are not used in the routine ECG interpretation. The axes of T wave and P wave are also not routinely determined. However, in the computer interpretation in modern electrocardiogram tracings the axes of P and T waves are now easily available. Thus, routine consideration of T and P wave axes is possible and may be helpful. T wave axis is discussed later in Section 5.3. The normal mean manifest *frontal plane P wave axis is also directed generally within the region of +40° to +60°* [2] *with the normal limits between 0° and +75°* [6]. The axis of P wave is affected by different conditions [2, 6], for example,

- +60° to +90° or even more to right axis deviation in acquired right heart diseases including due to chronic obstructive pulmonary disease (COPD) with tall upright P wave in II, aVF, and III leads with near equiphasic or equiphasic P waves in lead I,
- +45° to –30° in left atrial diseases with upright in I and aVL leads, and
- –80° to –90° in the retrograde activation of the atria by an impulse from AV node or below with inverted P wave in II, aVF, and III leads.

4.4. Usefulness and limitations of the computer interpretations in modern electrocardiograms

The computer interpretations in modern electrocardiogram tracings help to note if anything is missed or to crosscheck the findings. But that does not decrease the responsibility of the physicians. In the textbook on electrocardiogram prepared on behalf of the council on clinical cardiology of the American Heart Association, it is emphasized: "*Even though computer interpretations of ECGs are readily available, the clinician's role as overseer and final interpreter has not and must not be diminished*" [9]. On the other hand, one should also not totally ignore the computer interpretations. The computer interpretations are particularly useful for *rate, axes of QRS, P and T waves, intervals and amplitude, or voltage and duration of different waves*. Though in the computer interpretation the range of normal values is not given, the possible abnormal findings are indicated. The overall computer interpretation in the modern electrocardiogram machines, however, cannot incorporate the various clinical conditions to be considered in each individual patient. The rhythm, P, QRS, and T wave morphology, and ST segment need to be given particular attention by the clinicians and the conclusion should be drawn considering all the clinical conditions of the individual patient.

5. Effect of axis deviation on QRS-T morphology

5.1. Variations in the QRS pattern and usually negative waves in aVR

The QRS pattern in the extremity leads may vary considerably from one normal subject to another depending on the electrical axis of the QRS, which describes the mean orientation of the QRS vector with reference to the six frontal plane leads [16]. The effects on QRS and T morphologies by different frontal plane QRS axes may thus cause confusion in the interpretation of ECG. A shift, even a pronounced one, of the heart to the right due to pneumothorax or pleural effusion, however, does not necessarily affect the frontal plane QRS axis [17]. The effect of axis in the QRS and T morphologies can also be utilized for the efficient interpretation of electrocardiogram. The frontal plane QRS axis in most people are directed away from aVR, thus in the lead aVR the QRS complex is mostly negative. Marked left axis (<–60°) or right axis (>+120°) or extreme axis deviation will cause positive QRS complex in aVR. And the dominantly upright QRS as well as P waves in aVR along with the inverted ones in leads I and aVL indicate the presence of reversal of the left and right arm electrodes or rarely the dextrocardia, a common form of cardiac malposition [2, 18]. Thus, while interpreting any ECG it is helpful to look first at aVR to quickly detect the incorrectly placed arm electrodes or the marked left or right axis deviation.

5.2. An example of the effect on QRS complex due to left axis deviation

The ECG with the recordings of the limb leads shown in **Figure 5** is used as an example to discuss the effect of left axis deviation on the appearance of QRS complex. In the ECG shown in **Figure 5**, the QRS complexes in III and aVF appear mostly negative raising the possibility of inferior wall ischemia. But this pattern in the asymptomatic person is most likely due to the frontal plane mean axis being at around –40°. The equiphasic points for this mean axis of –40° are at right angle, that is, at +50° and at –130°. The leads aVF and III are away from the equiphasic point at +50° toward the opposite pole of mean axis in the "*negative-half area of the mean axis*" (**Figure 3**) and are recording the increasingly negative QRS complex. Thus, the QRS complexes in III and aVF appear mostly negative. An ECG with right axis deviation is similarly likely to cause predominantly negative QRS complex in the leads I and aVL.

5.3. An example of the effect on T wave due to left axis deviation

Similarly the T waves in leads aVF and III in the ECG in **Figure 3** appear flat or inverted raising the possibility of inferior wall ischemia. However, as a rule the mean T wave axis and the mean QRS axis normally point in the same general (but not identical) direction [5]. Thus, in general when the main QRS deflection is positive (upright), the T wave is normally also positive [5] and vice versa. *In the adult, the QRS-T angle normally does not exceed 45° in the frontal plane [6]. When the angle is greater than 60°, the electrocardiogram is abnormal and disease is usually present [2].* In the ECG in **Figure 5**, the mean axis is directed at around –40° with the QRS complexes in III and aVF appearing more negative. In the asymptomatic person with this ECG, the mean frontal plane T wave axis is likely to be directed as the mean frontal plane QRS axis with the T wave appearing flat or inverted like the QRS complex. The T wave axis given in the computer interpretation in the modern electrocardiogram may provide additional information to correlate with the clinical condition of the patient.

5.4. The variations in the QRS-T pattern and its implications

The mean axis of the QRS complex causing the variations in the QRS-T pattern is just one of the many factors to do so. Minor degrees of or apparent ST segment or T wave changes can also occur due to many general medical or cardiac conditions other than the ischemic ones. Various such conditions related to each individual patient are not incorporated in the computer interpretation of the ECG tracing. The clinician has to correlate the ECG findings with the clinical conditions of the patient.

The US Preventive Services Task Force (USPTF) recommends against screening with resting or exercise ECG for the prediction of coronary heart disease events in asymptomatic adults at low risk for coronary heart disease events. The USPSTF concludes that the current evidence is insufficient to assess the balance of benefits and harms of screening with resting or exercise ECG for the prediction of coronary heart disease events in asymptomatic adults at intermediate or high risk for coronary heart disease events [19]. The overall risk for a serious adverse event, one that requires hospitalization or causes sudden death, with exercise ECG is estimated to be up to 1 in 10,000 tests [20].

Moreover, up to 71% of asymptomatic adults with abnormal exercise treadmill ECG results have no angiographically demonstrable coronary artery stenosis [21] and revascularization as such has also not been shown to reduce coronary heart disease events in asymptomatic persons [19]. And the risk for any serious adverse event from angiography is up to 1.7%, including risk for death (0.1%), myocardial infarction (0.05%), stroke (0.07%), or arrhythmia

(0.4%) [19, 22]. Such complications are more likely in the countries where the skills of angiography and angioplasty are not certified with appropriate criteria (considering *the learning curve* required for the particular skill) and in the situation where *the volume of the procedures* performed by the operator or in the institutions are not sufficient.

6. Causes of left axis deviation

The conditions which are likely to fulfill the criteria of the defined cut-off points and are conventionally considered as the causes of left axis deviation [1, 2, 4–8, 17] are shown in **Table 1**. An individual patient may have more than one medical condition; in such conditions, the resultant axis deviation may not reflect the typical pattern of one cause.

Axis deviation in conditions like right bundle branch block (RBBB) and left bundle branch block (LBBB) also depends on their underlying causes. LBBB is commonly a sign of organic heart disease [2] and most patients with LBBB have underlying left ventricular hypertrophy [5]. Thus, left axis deviation is usually seen in LBBB. Though LBBB is even emphasized to be always a sign of heart disease usually of the left ventricle [7], it is rarely seen in normal individuals without any organic heart disease [5]. Some other congenital heart diseases where left axis deviation is seen include

- tricuspid atresia,
- single ventricle,
- congenitally corrected transposition of the great arteries, and
- double outlet right ventricle with infracristal ventricular septal defect [17].

- Left anterior fascicular block (left anterior hemiblock) (see **Table 2**)
- Inferior wall myocardial infarction
- Left ventricular hypertrophy due to various causes
- Left bundle branch block (see text)
- Ventricular tachycardia from a focus in the apex of the left ventricle
- Pacing from the apex of the right or left ventricle
- Primum atrial septal defect and endocardial cushion defect
- Other congenital heart diseases (see text)
- Wolff-Parkinson-White (WPW) syndrome: Less common type (previously called type B) affecting the right-sided accessory bypass pathways
- Hyperkalemia
- Emphysema and chronic obstructive pulmonary disease in about 10% (see text)

Table 1. Causes of left axis deviation.

In chronic obstructive pulmonary disease (COPD) with development of pulmonary hypertension, the frontal plane QRS axis shifts to the right side, even to +150° [2]. In very severe cases, extreme axis deviation may occur. Occasionally, in about 10% cases, there may be left axis deviation, the frontal plane QRS axis being directed upwards and to the left in the vicinity of –60° to –90° [2]. The exact mechanism is uncertain, but it is also supposed to be *an axis illusion* and the term *pseudo-left axis deviation* has also been applied [17]. In an individual patient with COPD, the presence of left axis deviation rather points out the need to look for other conditions, especially coronary heart disease, due to the common etiological factor of smoking shared by both diseases.

7. The leftward shift of axis

While enumerating the causes of axis deviation there may be confusion to

- whether the conditions mentioned are just likely to shift the axis toward one or other side of the usual normal axis between +40° and +60° (**Figure 2**) but within the conventionally considered limits or
- whether the conditions mentioned shift the axis frankly toward the right or left side fulfilling the defined limits of the axis deviations.

There are different physiological and pathological conditions which may shift the axis to one side or the other.

7.1. Effect of breathing

When a person breathes in, the diaphragm descends and the heart becomes more vertical and QRS electrical axis generally shifts toward right side, and when the person breathes out, the diaphragm ascends, heart assumes a more horizontal position, and the axis shifts toward the left side [5]. This may be more pronounced in maximum inspiration and expiration.

7.2. Body habitus and obesity

The mean frontal plane electrical axis also depends on body habitus [3]. The axes are more vertical in thin individuals and more horizontal in heavy individuals [6]. Obesity may deviate the frontal plane QRS axis toward the left side but not further to the left than 0° and a left axis deviation to –30° or further leftwards in an obese person probably represents a pathological abnormality [2, 23].

7.3. Pregnancy

A small rightward QRS axis shift may occur in the first trimester [24]. Similarly, some degree of leftward shift of QRS axis by about 15–30° has been reported in the third trimester of pregnancy by different studies [24–26] and the axis shifting back to normal side after delivery [26].

However, in some cases of pregnancy, a slight rightward shift of QRS axis (within the normal range) may occur at full term [27]. It is emphasized that pregnancy is not associated with left axis deviation or any significant change of QRS axis [2]. Thus, in general some degree of leftward shift of QRS axis may occur in the third trimester of pregnancy. However, an isolated rightward QRS axis change may be encountered in normal pregnant patients and cannot be viewed as a definite abnormality or used as a sole criterion for heart disease [24].

7.4. The causes of left axis deviation

The conditions which are likely to fulfill the criteria of the defined cut-off points and are conventionally considered as the causes of left axis deviation [1, 2, 4–8, 17] (**Table 1**) may also not fulfill the defined criteria especially in the initial stages but they may shift the axis to one side from its usual range of the degrees between +40° and +60° (**Figure 2**). Most causes of left axis deviation (**Table 1**) are well-known clinical entities. Isolated left axis deviation and leftward shift of axis have been increasingly noticed by the author especially in relatively young adults with diabetes. There are many points to consider regarding leftward shift of axis and particularly the isolated left anterior fascicular block.

8. The isolated left anterior fascicular conduction delay

There are different causes of left axis deviation (**Table 1**). Left axis deviation may also occur in the absence of apparent cardiac disease and it is not necessarily a sign of significant underlying heart disease [5]. Left axis deviation is relatively common with advancing age even in the absence of clinically overt heart disease and rare during early adult years [17, 28–40]. In a population-based study of the people 20 years and above, almost half of the people with left axis deviation had isolated left axis deviation without evidence of heart diseases [28]. Left anterior fascicular block is the most common cause of left axis deviation [2]. The classical criteria of left anterior fascicular block are frontal plane axis between –45° and –90°, qR pattern in lead aVL, R peak time in lead aVL of 45 ms or more, and QRS duration less than 120 ms [3]. There are different causes of left anterior fascicular block or conduction delay [2, 5, 17, 27] (**Table 2**). In neuromuscular diseases like myotonia dystrophica, the involvement appears to be in the cardiac conduction system as a sort of nonmyopathic manifestations [17]. Hyperkalemia as well as a sudden increase in serum potassium levels are sometimes accompanied by left axis deviation ascribed to left anterior fascicular block due to changes in resting membrane potential and transmembrane potassium gradient; similar mechanism is held responsible for the generalized QRS widening with hyperkalemia [17].

The finding of isolated left anterior fascicular block is a very common, nonspecific abnormality [5]. The QRS axes which range from 0° to –30° probably reflect minor degrees of left anterior fascicular block or incomplete left anterior fascicular block [2]. An axis of +29° is also considered as already reflecting some degree of left axis deviation [2]. Complete block of conduction in the left anterior fascicle is not necessary to produce left axis deviation; presumably, all that is required

Clinical cardiac diseases	Other conditions
• Coronary heart disease • Left ventricular hypertrophy • Chronic cardiac failure • Cardiomyopathies • Aortic valve diseases • Various congenital heart diseases • Cardiac surgery (especially aortic valve surgery) • Infiltrative diseases • Focal pathological lesions	• Ageing • Atherosclerosis • Long-standing hypertension • Other secondary degenerative disorders of the conduction system • Primary sclerodegenerative disorders, for example, Lenegre disease or Lev disease • Congenital isolated left anterior fascicular block • Neuromuscular diseases like myotonia dystrophica, peroneal muscular atrophy, limb-girdle dystrophy • Rarely in hyperkalemia

Table 2. Causes of left anterior fascicular block or conduction delay.

is enough delay in anterior fascicular conduction to result in the activation of the anterior left ventricular solely via the posterior fascicle [17]. In fascicular block, left axis deviation can be interpreted as either delayed conduction or complete block in the left anterior fascicle [17], which may explain the leftward shift of axis from minor degrees to frank left axis deviation.

9. Vulnerability of left anterior fascicle

The left anterior fascicle is more vulnerable to interruption than the left posterior fascicle because of many reasons [2, 17] (**Table 3**). The left anterior fascicle is often supplied by septal branch of descending artery only or by septal branch of descending artery and atrioventricular node artery or rarely by atrioventricular node artery alone [17]. A total occlusion of the left anterior descending artery may cause a subsequent right bundle branch block with left anterior fascicular block [1]. This is one of the reasons for the frequent manifestation of right bundle branch block with left anterior fascicular block [2].

	Left anterior fascicle	Left posterior fascicle
Length and width	Relatively long and thin	Relatively short and thick
Blood supply	Mostly single blood supply (see text)	Dual blood supply
Proximity to aortic valve	Closer (so likely to be affected by aortic valve disease and surgery)*	Further away from aortic valve*

*Left anterior fascicle is situated superiorly and left posterior fascicle inferiorly.

Table 3. Reasons of left anterior fascicular being more vulnerable to interruption than the left posterior fascicle.

10. Isolated left anterior fascicular conduction delay due to atherosclerosis and degenerative conditions

The causes and clinical significance of left axis deviation have always been of interest since the early days of electrocardiography [17]. In regards to the causation of isolated left anterior fascicular delayed conduction or block, the possible mechanisms are fibrosis related to atherosclerosis and degenerative conditions [17]. The vulnerability of left anterior fascicle to interruption (**Table 3**) indicates the possibility of atherosclerosis with resultant coronary heart diseases. The possibility has, thus, been pointed out that left anterior fascicular block which occurs in the elderly may be due to subclinical coronary artery disease [2]. Ischemic heart disease in its own right causes fibrosis that partially or completely interrupts conduction in one or more fascicles [17]. On the other hand, fibrosis and degenerative disorder of the anterior fascicle of left bundle branch are postulated to be the cause of left axis deviation in the older population without associated cardiovascular abnormalities [17, 37–41]. The ECG trend of the gradual leftward migration of the frontal QRS axis has been concluded to be a common sequel of aging, independent of the population prevalence of coronary atherosclerosis. Thus, isolated, age-related degenerative disease is also considered to cause a variety of infranodal conduction defects that are unrelated to coexisting myocardial disease or coronary artery obstruction, which may be negligible or absent [17].

Interatrial conduction block by fibrosis: It is interesting to note here that the association between conduction delays and block in Bachmann's bundle (**Figure 5**) and atrial fibrillation has been reported [42]. The Bachmann's bundle is recognized as a muscular bundle and shares electrophysiological properties of both Purkinje and atrial fibers; it is not surrounded by a fibrous tissue sheath. Fibrosis of the interatrial tract or Bachmann's bundle has been suggested as the mechanism underlying interatrial conduction block. Areas of conduction block may not be confined to Bachmann's bundle alone [42]. The association of such changes with the left axis deviation and left anterior fascicular conduction delay deserves study.

11. Left axis deviation and glucose intolerance

In a study of almost the entire population aged 16 years and above in a town in 1959–1960 among people with left axis deviation, more than 25%, and among those less than 40 years of age, 36–40%, have hyperglycemia with blood glucose value above the 80th percentile for the age group [32]. Similarly, in another study of people with diabetes and control group, diabetic men have more leftward frontal QRS axis than their nondiabetic counterparts when the effect of confounding factors (age, obesity, coronary heart disease, hypertension, and drugs) was taken into account [43]. In a population study, among people with isolated left axis deviation almost half (47.4%) of the persons less than 40 years age have blood glucose in the upper quintile values in comparison to 20.7% of those more than 50 years [28]. In a study of asymptomatic people aged 30 years or more not on any medication attending outdoor clinics for health checkup, the mean (SD) values of fasting plasma glucose are 101.0 ± 18.3 mg/dL in the slight left axis deviation group with QRS axis 0° to –30° (mean age 40.3 ± 8.5) and 122.9 ± 27.5 mg/dL in moderate-to-marked left axis deviation group with QRS axis –30° to –90° (mean age 54.5 ± 6.3). The frequency of glucose intolerance is 48.9% in the slight left axis deviation group with QRS axis 0° to –30° and 84.9% in moderate-to-marked left axis deviation group with QRS axis –30° to –90°, the difference being significant after conditioning the effects of age and sex ($P \leq 0.03$) and after conditioning the effect of BP ($P = 0.02$) [44, 45]. In a recent study with 85% of participants less than 55 years of age, left axis deviation was present in 8% of control group and 43.3% of type 2 diabetes [46]. The frequency of left axis deviation in the control nondiabetic group mostly below the age of 55 years in this report is also relatively high. The control group, though do not have diabetes, may have higher level of glucose or glycated hemoglobin (HbA1c) which could be related to the increasing glucose intolerance in the population now.

12. Why glucose intolerance as a cause of left anterior fascicular conduction delay was not much reported in earlier reports?

12.1. Difficulty in conducting fasting and 2-hour glucose estimation for diagnosis in the studies

In many reports of different findings in ECG of varied populations, plasma glucose estimation was mostly not done [29, 31, 33–40]. Conducting fasting and 2-hour glucose estimation in the field situation may not be easy as people have to come in the fasting state and wait for further 2 hours after taking glucose. Glycated hemoglobin (HbA1c) has been recently recommended for diagnosis of glucose intolerance.

12.2. A relatively new phenomenon

The epidemic of glucose intolerance in the world is relatively a new phenomenon starting since the latter half of twentieth century [47, 48]. It is now increasingly affecting the younger population [47]. The situation of the epidemic of diabetes could have led to observe and report the association of glucose intolerance and left axis deviation in relatively younger people more explicitly now [45, 46].

12.3. Data collection only as the normal axis or as the left axis deviation mostly with –30° to –90°

In most studies, including that of people with hyperglycemia or diabetes, only the presence of left axis deviation with QRS frontal plane axis –30° to –90° is considered [29–34, 36–39, 49], not the leftward shift of axis from its usual normal position (**Figure 2**), and thus the lower range of leftward shift is likely to be missed. The process of gradual shifting of the ECG axis toward left could be associated with the period of exposure to different grades and combination of the related factors like increasing age, glucose level, and other factors. Focusing only on the left axis deviation criteria as –30° to –90° by the studies also appears as one reason of dearth of evidences about the association of different degrees of QRS axis with possible factors. The arbitrary limits of the axis deviations have already been discussed.

13. Left axis deviation in school children in indigenous population

High prevalence of left axis deviation, 6–9-fold higher than the control group, in healthy American-Indian Navajo and Apache school children has been reported, the possible cause of which was considered unexplained [50]. Mean frontal plane QRS axis between –1° and –90° was present in 19% of the Navajo and 12% of the Apache school children. The prevalence of the lesser degree of leftward shift of axis is also likely to be higher. Even the lesser degree of leftward shift of axis is also quite significant in children as compared to adults, as the normal QRS axis is more on the right in children. For example, in the neonate the normal frontal plane QRS axis is between +60° and +190°, and the axis then shifts to the left and by ages 1–5 years, it is generally between +10° and +110°. Between 5 and 8 years of age, the normal QRS axis may extend to +140°, and between ages 8 and 16 years, the range of normal QRS extends to +120° [3]. The indigenous populations like the American-Indian are the ones who are affected the most since the middle of the twentieth century by the global diabetes epidemic [47, 48], and there is high prevalence of diabetes in the American-Indian indigenous population affecting even children [47, 51]. The high prevalence of leftward shift of axis in the children in such population is most likely related to the glucose intolerance which needs to be studied.

14. Brain white matter hyperintensities and left anterior fascicular block similarly related to glucose intolerance

White matter of the brain consists mostly of glial cells and myelinated axons for the transmission of neuronal electrical activity. With the wide availability of magnetic resonance imaging, there is often incidental discovery of white matter lesions appearing as hyperintensities on T2 weighted image [52, 53]. Pathological findings in the regions of white matter hyperintensities include myelin pallor, tissue rarefaction associated with loss of myelin and axons, and mild gliosis [52]. The factors associated with the brain white matter hyperintensities include ageing, hypertension, and diabetes [52, 53], as in the case of left anterior fascicular block. It may be relevant to note here that neuropathy, including the autonomic one, is a well-known common complication of diabetes and it may also be linked with, for example, as a later clinical manifestation of, white matter hyperintensities. A new study shows that even the impaired fasting glycemia, with the fasting plasma glucose below the diabetic range, is associated with a higher burden of brain white matter hyperintensities [54]. Among the people with isolated left axis deviation almost half of the persons less than 40 years of age have blood glucose in the upper quintile values [28]. Left anterior fascicle is similarly involved in the *transmission of cardiac electrical activity* and its vulnerability to the interruption (**Table 3**) could make it likely to be susceptible to oxidative injury due to the accumulation of various metabolic products of hyperglycemia.

Hyperglycemia is associated with fibrodegeneration of the left anterior fascicle, brain white matter, and other tissues. Chronic hyperglycemia affects various growth factors including fibroblast, collagen, fibronectin, contractile proteins, and extracellular matrix proteins in the body through different mechanisms. The various possible mechanisms of hyperglycemia leading to complications include nonenzymatic glycosylation, polyol pathway, abnormal microvascular blood flow, thickening and leakage of basement membrane of blood vessels, formation of reactive oxygen species, formation of vascular endothelial growth factors, and overproduction of superoxide by the mitochondrial electron chain [11, 12, 55]. Ageing associated with the fibrodegeneration of various tissues also involves insulin signaling pathways, reactive oxygen species, and oxidative damage at number of sites [55]. The final pathways of mechanism of complications and fibrodegeneration of various tissues due to hyperglycemia and ageing appear similar. Ageing is a known risk factor of glucose intolerance. And looking at the similar final pathways of mechanisms of complications and fibrodegeneration of the tissues in hyperglycemia and ageing, there could also be reciprocal relation between the two conditions.

15. Future perspectives—from research and public health point of views

From the point of view of leftward shift of axis, correlation of various degrees of frontal plane QRS axis (not just the presence or absence of left axis deviation) with fasting and 2-hour glucose and/or glycated hemoglobin levels

- in the general population [45],
- in the children of the indigenous population where left axis is observed [50], and
- in the people with higher brain white matter hyperintensities [52–54] (along with magnetic resonance imaging of heart and/or nerve conduction studies and/or tests of autonomic neuropathy)

will help to provide further evidences and thus to correlate various factors with leftward shift of axis and glucose intolerance. The value of research lies in its utility. In the situation of pandemic of glucose intolerance also affecting the leftward shift of axis in younger population, to utilize the already available evidences especially of the risk of obesity or glucose intolerance in the offspring of mother with obesity or with undernutrition [56], the control programs to protect the susceptible populations need to be implemented [47] (**Table 4**). In the background of inherent insulin resistance during pregnancy and increasing age of mothers, maintenance of the optimum prepregnancy weight in the population appears to the key in hand in the control program of diabetes epidemic [47]. This will also help to benefit the children of the indigenous population where the research on left axis deviation and diabetes has been conducted.

	Examples in the communicable disease	Possible examples in diabetes**
Prevention programs for individuals	• Immunization • Personal protective measures • Chemprophylaxis	• Primary prevention programs • Campaign and programs to help achieve by the people the recommended body mass index of the respective populations
Control programs to protect the other susceptible populations*	• Isolation • Quarantine • Vector control (e.g., mosquito control for various diseases, cyclops control for guinea worm, chicken and poultry culling for avian influenza) • Treatment of case (e.g., tuberculosis) and carrier	Campaign and programs for • Maintenance of optimal prepregnancy body weight, as per the recommended body mass index of the respective populations, especially in the affluent and/or urban parts of the societies and • Nutritional support for the girls and women of childbearing age in rural and poorer sections of the societies

*The vulnerable populations to be protected by the control program of diabetes include the offspring of malnourished or overweight mothers.

**National and international health and diabetes agencies should clearly spell out the control programs, with appropriate budget allocation, for control of diabetes epidemic to protect the progeny.

Table 4. Examples of prevention and control programs in the communicable diseases as a model for similar strategies for individuals and susceptible populations in diabetes epidemic.

16. Conclusion

The frontal plane QRS axis and especially the left axis deviation have always been the areas of interest in electrocardiogram. There are different physiological and pathological conditions which affect the axis and the axis shift itself also affects the QRS and ST morphologies. The approximate degree of axis can be easily determined by observing the electrocardiogram. Most causes of left axis deviation are well-known clinical entities. Isolated left axis deviation and leftward shift of the axis have increasingly been reported to be possibly associated with glucose intolerance. There are reasons why such association was previously not reported. The left anterior fascicle is as such vulnerable to interruption. The possible relation of glucose intolerance with brain white matter hyperintensities and even ageing also indicate the need to conduct research in these areas. However, the already available evidences should also be simultaneously utilized to protect the susceptible population. The bottom line of the frontal plane QRS axis is to record the actual degrees of the axes (not just the presence or absence of normal axis or left, right, or extreme axis deviations) and correlate the changes in the degrees of axis with the levels of the various possible factors in the individual patient or the study populations.

Author details

Madhur Dev Bhattarai

Address all correspondence to: mdb@ntc.net.np

Nepal Diabetes Association, Kathmandu, Nepal

References

[1] Dubin D. Rapid Interpretation of EKGs. 6th ed. Tampa: Cover Publishing Co; 2000

[2] Narasimhan C, Franchis J. Leo Shamroth—An Introduction to Electrocardiography. 8th ed. New Delhi: Wiley; 2013

[3] Surawicz B, Childers R, Deal BM, Gettes LS. AHA/ACCF/HRS recommendations for the standardization and interpretation of the electrocardiogram Part III: Intraventricular conduction disturbances. Circulation. 2009;**119**:e235-e240

[4] Prutkin JM. Basic principles of ECG analysis. UpToDate. 2017, Feb

[5] Goldberger Z, Shvilkin A, Goldberger AL. Goldberger's Clinical Electrocardiography—A Simplified Approach. 8th ed. Philadelphia: Elsevier/Saunders; 2013

[6] Wegner GS, Strauss DG. Marriott's Practical Electrocadiography. 12th ed. New Delhi: Wolters Kluwer Health/Lippincott Williams and Wilkins; 2014

[7] Hampton JR. The ECG Made Easy. 8th ed. Edinburg: Elsevier/Churchill Livingstone; 2013

[8] Goldman MJ. Principles of Clinical Electrocardiography. 11th ed. California: Lange Medical Publications/Maruzen Asia; 1982

[9] Akhtar M (Prepared on behalf of the Council on Clinical Cardiology of the American Heart Association). Examination of the Heart—The Electrocardiogram. Dallas: American Heart Association; 1990

[10] Blackburn H, Keys A, Simonson E, Rautharju P, Punsar S. The electrocardiographic in population studies—A classification system. Circulation. 1960;**21**:1160-1175

[11] Kumar, Clark. Kumar and Clark's Clinical Medicine. 9th ed. Edinburgh: Elsevier; 2017. pp. 944-947, 1264-1273

[12] Waugh A, Grant A. Ross and Wilson's Anatomy and Physiology in Health and Illness. 11th ed. Edinburgh: Churchill Livingstone/Elesevier; 2010. pp. 80-83

[13] Sauer WH. Left anterior fascicular block. UpToDate. 2017

[14] Pryour, Weaver, Blount. Electrocardiographic observations of 493 residents living at high altitude (10,150 feet). American Journal of Cardiology. 1965;**16**(4):494-499

[15] Raynaud, Valeix, Drouet, Escourrou, Durand. Electrocardiographic observations in high altitude residents of Nepal and Bolivia. International Journal of Biometerology. 1981;**25**(3):205-217

[16] Kasper DL, Fauchi AS, Hauser SL, Longo DL, Jameson JL, Loscalzo J. Harrisons' Principles of Internal Medicine. 19th ed. New York: McGraw Hill Education; 2015. pp. 1450-1459, 1481, 2423-2430

[17] Perloff JK, Roberts NK, Cabeen WR. Left axis deviation: A reassessment. Circulation. 1979;**60**(1):12-21

[18] Eldridge J, Richley D, Egglett C. Clinical Guidelines by Consensus: Recording a Standard 12-lead Electrocardiogram. London: Society for Cardiological Science and Technology; 2017

[19] Mayer VA (on behalf of the US Preventive Services Task Force). Screening for coronary heart disease with electrocardiography: U.S. Preventive Services Task Force Recommendation Statement. Annals of Internal Medicine. 2012;**157**:7

[20] Myers J, Arena R, Franklin B, Pina I, Kraus WE, McInnis K, et al. American Heart Association Committee on Exercise, Cardiac Rehabilitation, and Prevention of the Council on Clinical Cardiology, the Council on Nutrition, Physical Activity, and Metabolism, and the Council on Cardiovascular Nursing. Recommendations for clinical exercise laboratories: A scientific statement from the American Heart Association. Circulation. 2009;**119**:3144-3161. [PMID: 19487589]

[21] Hopkirk JA, Leader S, Uhl GS, Hickman Jr JR, Fischer J. Limitation of exercise-induced R wave amplitude changes in detecting coronary artery disease in asymptomatic men. Journal of the American College of Cardiology. 1984;**3**:821-826. [PMID: 6693653]

[22] Noto Jr TJ, Johnson LW, Krone R, Weaver WF, Clark DA, Kramer Jr JR, et al. Cardiac catheterization 1990: A report of the Registry of the Society for Cardiac Angiography and Interventions (SCA&I). Catheterization and Cardiovascular Diagnosis. 1991;**24**:75-83. [PMID: 1742788]

[23] Zack PM, Wiens RD, Kennedy HL. Left axis deviation and adiposity: The US Health and Nutrition Examination Survey. The American Journal of Cardiology. 1984;**53**:1129

[24] Wegner NK. The ECG in normal pregnancy. Archives of Internal Medicine. 1982;**142**:1088

[25] Madras V, Challa N. Electrocardiographic variations during three trimesters of normal pregnancy. International Journal of Research in Medical Sciences. 2015;**3**(9):2218-2222

[26] Goloba M, Nelson S, Macfarlane. The electrocardiogram in pregnancy. Computing in Cardiology. 2010;**37**:693-696

[27] Schwartz DB, Schamroth L. The effect of pregnancy on the frontal plane QRS axis. Journal of Electrocardiology. 1979;**12**:1129

[28] Ostrander LD. Left axis deviation: Prevalence, associated conditions, and prognosis: An epidemiological study. Annals of Internal Medicine. 1971;**75**(1):23-28

[29] Kitchin AH, Lowther CP, Milne JS. Prevalence of clinical and electrocardiographic evidence of ischaemic heart disease in the older population. British Heart Journal. 1973;**35**(9):946-953

[30] de Bacquer D, de Baker G, Kornitzer M. Prevalences of ECG findings in large population based samples of men and women. Heart. 2000;**84**(6):625-633

[31] Lakkireddy DR, Clark RA, Mohiuddin SM. Electrocardiographic findings in patients>100 years of age without clinical evidence of cardiac disease. The American Journal of Cardiology. 2003;**92**(10):1249-1251

[32] Ostrander LD, Brandt RL, Kjelsberg MO, Epstein FH. Electrocardiographic findings among the adult population of a natural community, Tecumseh, Michigan. Circulation. 1965;**31**:888-898

[33] Hingorani P, Natekar M, Deshmukh S, Karnad DR, Kothari S, Narula D, Lokhandwala Y. Morphological abnormalities in baseline ECGs in healthy normal volunteers participating in phase I studies. The Indian Journal of Medical Research. 2012;**135**:322-330

[34] Hiss RG, Lamb LE. Electrocardiographic findings in 122,043 individuals. Circulation. 1962;**25**:947-961

[35] Mason JW, Ramseth DJ, Chanter DO, Moon TE, Goodman DB, Mendzelevski B. Electrocardiographic reference ranges derived from 79,743 ambulatory subjects. Journal of Electrocardiology. 2007;**40**(3):228-234

[36] Bahl OP, Walsh TJ, Massie E. Left axis deviation: An electrocardiographic study with post-mortem correlation. British Heart Journal. 1969;**31**(4):451-456

[37] Grayzel J, Neyshaboori M, Paramw NJ. Left-axis deviation: Etiologic factors in one-hundred patients. American Heart Journal. 1975;**89**(4):419-427

[38] Corne RA, Beasmish RE, Rollwagen RL. Significance of left anterior hemiblock. British Heart Journal. 1978;**40**(5):552-557

[39] Grant RP. Left axis deviation: An electrocardiographic-pathological correlation study. Circulation. 1956;**14**(2):233-249

[40] Das G. Left axis deviation—A spectrum of intraventricular conduction block. Circulation. 1976;**53**(6):917-919

[41] Bradlow BA. The importance of abnormal left axis deviation in life assurance. South African Medical Journal. 1973:**47**(20):877-881

[42] van Campenhout MJH, Yaksh A, Kik C, de Jaegere PP, Yen S, Allessie MA, de Groot NMS. Bachmann's Bundle—A key player in the development of atrial fibrillation. Circulation Arrhythmia and Electrophysiology. 2013;**6**:1041-1046

[43] Uusitupa M, Mustonen J, Siitonen O, Pyorala K. Quantitative electrocardiographic and vectorcardiographic study on newly-diagnosed non-insulin-dependent diabetic and non-diabetic control subjects. Cardiology. 1988;**75**(1):1-9

[44] Paudyal A (under the guidance of Bhattarai MD). Correlation of normal QRS duration left axis deviation in ECG with clinical and investigation parameters in patients without cardiac symptoms [thesis for MD in Internal Medicine]. Kathmandu: National Academy of Medical Sciences; 2008

[45] Paudyal A, Bhattarai MD, Karki BB, Bajracharya MR, Rajouria AD, Pradhan A. Left axis deviation in electrocardiogram with normal QRS duration in ambulatory adults without cardiac symptoms: A possible marker of glucose intolerance. Journal of Nepal Medical Association. 2013;**52**(192):557-562. PMID: 25327226

[46] Helaihil AF, Hatim I, Abed AH. Isolated left axis deviation in diabetic patients. Journal of Pharmacy. 2015;**5**(3):36-45

[47] Bhattarai MD. Three patterns of rising type 2 diabetes prevalence in the world: need to widen the concept of prevention in individuals into control in the community. Journal of Nepal Medical Association. 2009;**48**(174):173-179. PMID: 20387365

[48] Bhattarai MD. Response to Donovan et al. Does exposure to hyperglycaemia in utero increase the risk of obesity and diabetes in the offspring. Diabetic Medicine. 2016;**33**:5. dme.12980. PMID:26435160

[49] Pfister R, Cairns R, Erdmann E, Schneider CA (on behalf of the PROactive investigators). Prognostic impact of electrocardiographic signs in patients with type 2 diabetes and cardiovascular diseases: Results from the PROactive study. Diabetic Medicine. 2011;**28**(10):1206-1212

[50] Ewy GA, Okada RD, Marcus FI, Goldberg SJ, Phibbs BP. Electrocardiographic axis deviation in Navajo and Apache Indians. Chest. 1979;**75**(1):54-58

[51] Gohdes D, Kaufman S, Valway S. Diabetes in American Indians: An overview. Diabetes Care. 1993;**16**(1):239-243

[52] Debette S, Markus HS. The clinical importance of white matter hyperintensities on brain magnetic resonance imaging: Systemic review and meta-analysis. British Medical Journal. 2010;**341**:c3666. PMID: 20660506

[53] Murray AD, Staff RT, Shenkin SD, Deary IJ, Starr JM, Whalley LJ. Brain white matter hyperintensities: Relative importance of vascular risk factors in nondemented elderly people. Radiology. 2005;**237**(1):251-257. PMID: 16126931

[54] White Matter Lesions Linked to Rising Plasma Glucose. Medscape. Atlanta: WebMD; Nov 24, 2015

[55] Walker BR, Colledge NR, Ralston SH, Penman ID. Davidson's Principles and Practice of Medicine. 22nd ed. Edinburgh: Elsevier/Churchill Livingstone; 2014. pp. 168-170, 532-534

[56] Ozanne SE, Constancia M. Mechanisms of disease: The developmental origin of disease and the role of the epigenotype. Nature Clinical Practice Endocrinology & Metabolism; 2007;**3**:539-546

Chapter 3

Signal-Averaged ECG: Basics to Current Issues

Ioana Mozos and Dana Stoian

Additional information is available at the end of the chapter

http://dx.doi.org/10.5772/intechopen.69279

Abstract

Signal-averaged ECG (SAECG) is a high-resolution, noninvasive electrocardiographic method enabling detection of late ventricular potentials (LVP), which are low-amplitude and high-frequency signals, predicting reentry ventricular arrhythmias, and sudden cardiac death (SCD). Three criteria are used to detect late ventricular potentials as follows: signal-average ECG QRS duration (SAECG-QRS), the duration of the terminal part of the QRS complex with an amplitude below 40 μV (LAS40) and the root mean square (RSM) signal amplitude of the last 40 ms of the signal < 20 μV (RMS40). Late ventricular potentials can be detected not only at the end of a QRS complex but also as intra-QRS (IQRS) potentials. Signal-averaged ECG was modified to enable the analysis of the P-wave and to detect atrial late potentials (ALPs), low-amplitude potentials at the terminal part of the filtered P-wave, and predictors of atrial fibrillation (AF). Late atrial and ventricular potentials originate from areas of delayed, fragmented, and heterogenous conduction within atrial or ventricular myocardium. This chapter reviews the most important mechanisms explaining the occurrence of late ventricular, intra-QRS, and atrial potentials; their predictive value for arrhythmia, focusing on recent clinical data, long-term follow-up, and outcome; and analysis of SAECG variables in cardiac and noncardiac diseases.

Keywords: late ventricular potentials, atrial late potentials, ventricular arrhythmia risk, atrial fibrillation

1. Introduction

Cardiovascular disorders are leading mortality causes worldwide. Prophylactic methods and early detection deserve special attention. The standard 12-lead electrocardiogram (ECG) is a simple, reliable, and cost-effective method, used in clinical practice and trials for sudden cardiac death (SCD) risk stratification, considering QT and QRS duration, fragmented QRS complexes, and Tpeak-tend interval. Signal-averaged ECG (SAECG) can detect very small, subtle signals (microvolt level), which are not visible when using standard 12-lead ECG, by averaging and filtering multiple ECG complexes [1–3]. The high-resolution or signal-averaged ECG has been recommended by the European Society of Cardiology, the American Heart Association, and the American College of Cardiology as a useful tool to improve the diagnosis and risk stratification of patients with ventricular arrhythmias or those at risk of developing life-threatening ventricular arrhythmias [4].

The substrate for SCD varies from advanced cardiomyopathic injuries, myocardial infarction scars to no obvious sign of structural damage [4]. The most common cause of SCD is coronary heart disease, but several cardiomyopathies, heart failure, and genetic influences, as well as myocarditis, pericardial diseases, pulmonary arterial hypertension, rheumatic disease, end-stage renal failure, endocrine disorders, obesity, anorexia, hypertension, lipid abnormalities, diabetes mellitus, several drugs, and physical and toxic agents can also be involved [4]. Several inherited abnormalities, including long and short QT interval, Brugada syndrome, and catecholaminergic ventricular tachycardia (VT), can precipitate SCD without any structural changes in the heart, triggered by external events [4].

Atrial fibrillation (AF) is the most frequent arrhythmia in the general population, with poorly understood underlying mechanisms of structural and electrical atrial remodeling [5]. It is associated with an increased risk of stroke, heart failure, and mortality [5].

The aim of this chapter is to review the most important mechanisms explaining the occurrence of late ventricular, intra-QRS (IQRS), and atrial potentials; their predictive value for arrhythmia, focusing on recent studies, long-term follow-up, and outcome; and analysis of SAECG variables in cardiac and noncardiac diseases.

2. Late ventricular potentials

LVPs are low-amplitude, high-frequency signals, occurring in the terminal part of the QRS complex, as markers of electrophysiological cardiac substrates for reentry ventricular arrhythmia, favored by structural heterogeneity due to myocardial necrosis, fibrosis, or dystrophy [6]. LVPs appear if conduction is slow enough to enable reentry and a unidirectional block is present [6]. They assess ventricular depolarization, and the signal is more stable and reproducible than the repolarization process [6]. Arrhythmia triggers are autonomic imbalances (increased sympathetic activity), acute ischemia, or electrolyte disorders. Temporal and frequency domain analysis can be performed to detect arrhythmia risk.

Three criteria are used to detect LVPs as follows: SAECG-QRS duration , the duration of the terminal part of the QRS complex with an amplitude below 40 μV (LAS40), and the root mean square signal amplitude of the last 40 ms of the signal < 20 μV (RMS40) [7].

SAECG-QRS was considered prolonged if it exceeds 120 [7] or 114 ms according to other authors [8, 9]. LAS40 is pathological if exceeding 38 ms and RMS40 if less than 20 μV [7]. Late

http://dx.doi.org/10.5772/intechopen.69279

ventricular potentials are defined by the presence of one or two of the mentioned positive criteria (**Figures 1, 2**) [7, 10].

Considering their low amplitude, LVPs can only be detected if amplified, filtered, and averaged using high-resolution SAECG or body surface mapping. Electronic filters can further reduce signal noise by eliminating high-frequency signals such as skeletal muscle potentials [3]. The filters used in SAECG provide different numerical and diagnostic results, with a higher sensitivity for 40–250-Hz filters compared to 40-Hz filters [1]. The authors of the present chapter have experience only with 50–250 Hz filters. ECG signals are collected for 5–20 min, followed by averaging the QRS complexes through the temporal technique to reduce the signal-to-noise ratio [3].

The most important limitations in SAECG are related to electrical interference causing false results and the low positive predictive value for arrhythmic events [6, 11, 12]. However, they have a high negative predictive value for arrhythmic events [12]. Their presence predicts inducibility of ventricular tachycardia at invasive electrophysiology studies, and if they are combined with low ejection fraction, they enable detection of patients at high risk of sudden cardiac death [3].

Besides time-domain (TD) analysis of SAECG, frequency domain analysis may also provide valuable data. Abrupt changes in the frequency contents between adjacent overlapping segments of the QRS complex are the markers of the arrhythmogenic substrate in spectral turbulent analysis (STA) [13].

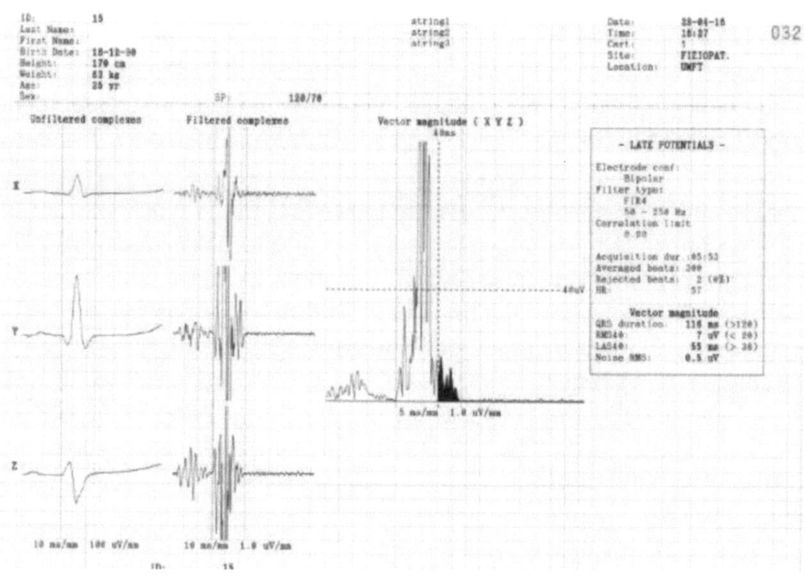

Figure 1. Late ventricular potentials with two positive criteria (LAS40 and RMS40).

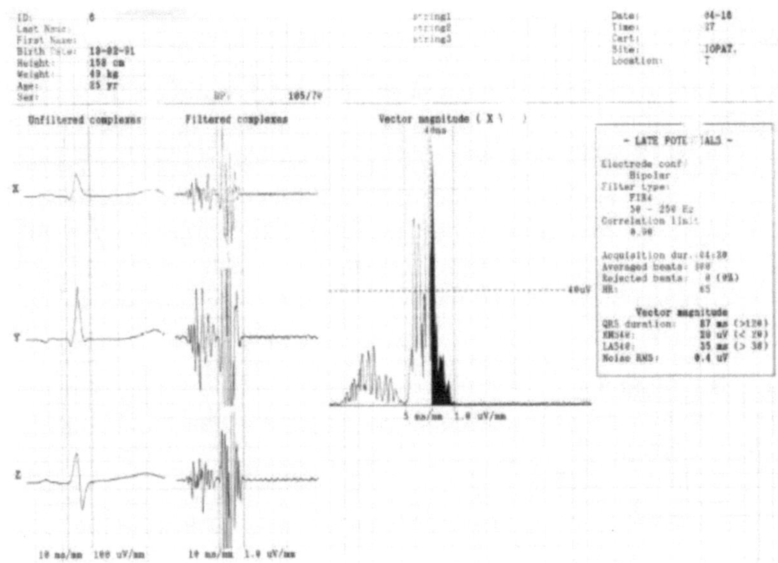

Figure 2. Normal SAECG and no late ventricular potentials.

The sensitivity of SAECG is higher compared to standard 12-lead ECG for identifying patients with acute coronary syndrome [14]. LVPs were initially used in patients with myocardial infarction. They appear in the heterogenous tissue at the border of a myocardial infarction scar [6], very frequent in nonseptal myocardial segments, and were abolished in most patients with myocardial infarction after ventricular tachycardia ablation, associated with scar homogenization and a low recurrence rate [15]. The utility of SAECG was questioned in the post-percutaneous coronary intervention era [3]. LVPs have been recorded in several other cardiac disorders, especially cardiomyopathies, myocarditis, infiltrative heart disease, arrhythmogenic right ventricular dysplasia, congenital heart defects, heart failure, left ventricular hypertrophy, Brugada syndrome, early repolarization, bundle branch block, and atrial fibrillation [6, 16–18]. Despite improved postinfarction survival due to lifestyle changes, thrombolytic, antiplatelet therapy, beta-blockers, and revascularization, LVPs can still be used in selecting patients for interventional studies [6]. Dinov et al. [19] found a positive correlation between endocardial scar area and filtered QRS in patients with ischemic VT, normalization of SAECG after catheter ablation (CA), and abnormal SAECG after CA as a predictor for VT recurrence (**Table 1**). Conduction delay contributed to ventricular dyssynchrony, regardless of LVPs in patients with heart failure, and LVPs did not play an important role in ventricular dyssynchrony [16]. Several SAECG studies have been performed in patients who underwent heart transplant [20–22]. SAECG distinguished between heart transplant patients with or without rejection, especially LAS40 and RMS40 [22]. The association between LVPs and rejection of heart transplant is explained by occurrence of areas of myocardial fibrosis, due to cell changes caused by alloreactive T lymphocytes against graft antigens and ischemia-reperfusion injuries as soon as the blood flow is reestablished [22].

http://dx.doi.org/10.5772/intechopen.69279

Study population	Results	Follow up	References
52 psychiatric patients 30 healthy controls	The prevalence of LVPs was significantly higher in psychiatric patients, not influenced by age, gender, and therapy	46 months, 3 SCD	Antoniou et al. [28]
50 patients with ischemic VT undergoing CA	A significant correlation was found between the surface SAECG and endocardial scar size in patients with ischemic VTs. A successful CA can result in normalization of SAECG and more favorable long-term outcomes. SAECG can predict the procedural success of VT ablation		Dinov et al. [19]
28 heart transplant patients	The presence of fibrosis with increased LAS40 and decreased RMS40 showed a good ability to distinguish between patients with and without rejection		Mendes et al. [22]
100 postmyocardial infarction patients undergoing electroanatomical mapping-based VT ablation	LVPs were abolished in 51% improving outcome		Tsiachris et al. [15]
41 patients with COPD and 63 patients without any history of pulmonary disease, matched for age and hypertension history	SAECG parameters and LVPs have little value in risk stratification for ventricular arrhythmias in COPD patients		Buzea et al. [27]
26 patients with newly diagnosed epilepsy, and no clinical evidence of heart disease were examined with SAECG and standard ECG. 15 patients were treated with lamotrigine and 10 with carbamazepine	Lack of antiepileptic drug-induced electrocardiographic abnormalities	3–9 months	Svalheim et al. [31]
45 patients with epilepsy and 19 healthy volunteers, younger than 46 years	Epilepsy patients more frequently display abnormal SAECGs with LVPs compared to the control group, and their presence correlates with the disease duration, refractory epilepsy, and polytherapy		Rejdak et al. [23]
64 patients with interventricular and intraventricular dyssynchronies	Filtered QRS duration provides more information to estimate ventricular dyssynchrony in patients with reduced ejection fraction than simple QRS duration; LVPs did not correlate with ventricular dyssynchrony		Tahara et al. [16]
20 young heart transplant patients	SAECG is not effective in detecting heart transplant rejection in young patients		Horenstein et al. [21]

Study population	Results	Follow up	References
70 acromegalic patients and 70 control subjects, age- and sex-matched	A higher prevalence of LVPs in acromegaly which significantly correlated with Lown scale of premature ventricular contractions		Maffei et al. [34]
48 patients with acromegaly: 16 active disease, 32 cured or 'well controlled', under treatment with sandostatin analogs, and 38 healthy volunteers	LVPs are frequently seen in active acromegaly as an early and sensitive parameter of myocardial injury		Herrmann et al. [36]

Table 1. LVP studies.

Extracardiac disorders were also associated with LVPs, especially hypertension, metabolic syndrome, obesity, eating disorders, diabetes mellitus, renal failure, chronic obstructive pulmonary disease (COPD), acromegaly, thalassemia, connective tissue diseases, epilepsy, and schizophrenia [6, 23–27]. Antiarrhythmic therapy, thrombolytic drugs, statins, steroids, and coronary interventions may influence LVPs [6].

Sudden cardiac death is higher in psychiatric patients, especially those with depression and schizophrenia than in the general population [28]. Several factors influence the relationship with cardiovascular disorders in patients with depression: social factors (poverty, social inequality, reduced access to healthcare), biological factors (endothelial dysfunction, impaired heart rate variability and platelet function, inflammation, hyperactivity of hypothalamic-pituitary-adrenal axis), higher prevalence of cardiovascular risk factors, and therapy (side effects of tricyclic, lower adherence) [29]. Both schizophrenia and depression impair the autonomic tone, ion channels, alter connexin 43 expression, and may cause drug-induced cardiac fibrosis [28].

Several factors enable ventricular arrhythmias in patients with epilepsy, such as sympathovagal imbalance, impaired cardiac repolarization, mutations of ionic channels affecting both the brain and the heart, dysfunctional cortical networks, ictal hypoxemia and hypercapnia, stress hormones, therapy, cardiorespiratory interactions, and associated cardiovascular diseases [24, 30]. Epilepsy patients more frequently displayed abnormal SAECGs with LVPs compared to healthy controls, correlated with disease duration, uncontrolled seizures, and polytherapy [23]. Svalheim et al. [31] reported no electrocardiographic changes (in standard ECG and SAECG) after antiepileptic drugs (carbamazepine and lamotrigene) in 26 epileptic patients.

COPD was associated with cardiovascular morbidity and mortality, considering negative cardiac effects of hyperinflation, exercise limitation, smoking, and hypoxemia [6]. Carjea found a higher prevalence of LVPs in patients with COPD, especially in moderate and severe cases [32]. Yildiz et al. [33] reported a significantly increased total QRS duration in patients with COPD compared to control subjects and LVPs but no significant association with premature ventricular contractions. Despite higher prevalence of LVPs, premature ventricular contractions, and complex ventricular arrhythmias in patients with COPD compared to healthy controls, SAECG had little value in stratification of ventricular arrhythmia risk in a study including 41 patients with COPD and 63 patients without any history of pulmonary disease [27].

Persistent, life-threatening ventricular arrhythmias may occur in several endocrine disorders, such as pheochromocytoma, acromegaly, primary aldosteronism, Addison disease, hypo- and hyperparathyroidism, and hypothyroidism [4]. Ventricular arrhythmias may occur due to excess or insufficient hormone activity on myocardial receptors, myocardial changes, electrolyte imbalances, or acceleration of progression of structural cardiac disorders [4]. Sudden death and increased prevalence of ventricular arrhythmias and LVPs have been described in acromegaly [34]. Ventricular arrhythmia risk in acromegaly is related to the specific cardiomyopathy associated with left ventricular hypertrophy, myocardial fibrosis, comorbidities, especially hypertension and sleep apnea, and, possibly, to the direct effects of the growth hormone and insulin growth factor 1 on myocardial cells and cardiac ion channels [34, 35]. The prevalence of LVPs was significantly higher in patients with acromegaly compared to healthy controls, related to a longer duration of the disease, premature ventricular contractions, and left ventricular hypertrophy [34]. Herrmann et al. [36] also reported LVPs in patients with active and well-controlled acromegaly, as a sensitive and early sign of myocardial injury, not related to muscle mass and body mass index, age, gender, and duration of the disease.

Thyroid hormone exerts several effects on the cardiovascular system [37]. Ventricular arrhythmia and sudden cardiac death may occur especially in hypothyroidism, probably related to prolonged QT interval [4]. LVPs have been described in hypo- and hyperthyroidism, according to a study including 278 patients with thyroid disorders even in subclinical dysfunctions [38]. A case of severe primary hypothyroidism was presented with an abnormal SAECG with LVPs, which disappeared with thyroxine therapy [37].

Future SAECG studies should also include patients with Cushing's syndrome, considering impaired cardiac function and structure due to the direct toxic effect of cortisol, increased blood pressure, central obesity, metabolic syndrome, hyperglycemia, and chronic hypokalemia [39]. Subclinical structural and functional cardiac alterations are very common but underdiagnosed [39].

3. Intra-QRS potentials

IQRSPs are low-amplitude notches (the order of microvolts), usually invisible in the standard ECG, which may occur anywhere in the signal-averaged QRS [2] and may not prolong the normal QRS duration [40]. They were described as the signals with sudden slope changes [40]. Extracting IQRSPs is challenging, considering that they are very weak signals, with abrupt changes in slope, approximation errors, and the differences among patients with ventricular arrhythmias [41]. The root mean square values were highly correlated with the parameters of the abnormal intra-QRS potentials in healthy controls but not in patients with ventricular tachycardia [40].

A combination of IQRSPs and LVPs can improve predictive accuracy for patients of high risk of ventricular arrhythmias.

4. P-wave potentials

P-wave signal-averaged electrocardiography, atrial late potentials (ALP), and abnormal intra-P-wave potentials could detect patients at risk of supraventricular arrhythmias, especially atrial fibrillation [42, 43]. ALP originates from areas of delayed and heterogenous conduction within the atrial myocardium, responsible for the occurrence of AF [44].

Prolonged filtered P-wave duration (FPD) in P-wave signal-averaged electrocardiography has been used as a noninvasive, powerful predictor of AF, the first episode and recurrences, in lone, occult or silent atrial fibrillation, in stroke, heart failure, hypertension, hypertrophic cardiomyopathy, hypothyroidism and in patients undergoing coronary artery bypass surgery [44–46]. A prolonged SAECG P-wave duration was also mentioned in septal atrial defect, especially in patients who experienced AF, not corrected after atrial septal defect closure, and it was demonstrated that atrial conduction disturbances occur early, requiring an early intervention to prevent the development of late AF (**Table 2**) [47].

There is no consensus about the cut-off point for FPD, which was 121 ms in hypertensive patients Auriti et al. [48], 124 ms in patients in sinus rhythm, 136 ms in hypertensive patients with a history of atrial fibrillation, 132 ms in patients with COPD, and 155 ms in several other studies [43, 45, 46, 49], differences related to different averaging and filtering methods [45].

Study population	Results	Follow up	References
45 patients with exacerbation of COPD and 58 age-matched patients with no history of pulmonary disease in a control group	The patients with acute exacerbation of COPD have a higher incidence of supraventricular arrhythmias. P-wave SAECG analysis has little value in the arrhythmic risk evaluation of these patients	Isolated atrial premature beats (APB) and supraventricular tachycardia (SVT)	Buzea et al. [43]
37 hypertensive patients with a first AF episode 37 age- and sex-matched hypertensive controls without AF	P-wave temporal and energy characteristics can identify hypertensive patients at risk of AF recurrence		Dakos et al. [50]
68 stroke patients in sinus rhythm, without history of AF	ALP is a novel predictor of AF in stroke patients. P-SAECG should be considered in stroke	11±4 months	Yodogawa et al. [44]
35 patients with atrial septal defect	Prolonged P-wave duration does not change after atrial septal defect closure	8±6 months after atrial septal defect closure	Thilen et al. [47]
4 generations kindred of 27 individuals, 8 with AF on the ECG	Persons with AF and mutation carriers (on chromosome 5p15) can be identified by a prolonged P-SAECG duration		Darbar et al. [49]
41 patients with two or more symptomatic episodes of idiopathic and persistent atrial fibrillation after successful electrical cardioversion and 25 healthy controls	Fragmented electrical activity, use of amiodarone, and positive terminal portion of the Z-lead of the P-SAECG were independent predictors of recurrence of idiopathic and persistent atrial fibrillation	6 months, 12 months, atrial fibrillation recurrences	Barbosa et al. [42]

Study population	Results	Follow up	References
101 patients in sinus rhythm before coronary artery bypass grafting (CABG)	The risk of AF after CABG can be predicted preoperatively with P-wave SAECG		Budeus et al. [46]
55 hypertensive patients with a history of atrial fibrillation 40 hypertensive patients without a history of atrial fibrillation.	Hypertensive patients with paroxysmal atrial fibrillation can be detected while in sinus rhythm by signal-averaged ECG P-wave duration		Aytemir et al. [45]

Table 2. Atrial late potentials (ALP) and fragmented electrical activity on the P-wave.

Besides FPD, Buzea et al. [43] also used the RMS voltages in the last 40, 30, and 20 ms of the filtered P-wave (RMS 40, RMS 30, and RMS 20), the root mean square voltage of the filtered P-wave potentials (RMS-p), and the integral of the potentials during the filtered P-wave (Integral-p), and defined ALP as FPD > 132 ms and RMS 20 < 2.3 μV.

Fragmentations are expected to occur throughout atrial depolarization and not only in its terminal part, and inter- and intra-atrial conduction may be impaired [42]. High-frequency fragmented electrical activity on the P-wave in patients with recurrent AF is the expression of atrial electrical heterogeneity, responsible for reentry circuits in the atria [42]. Barbosa et al. [42] used spectral turbulence analysis of the P-SAECG to detect abnormal intra-P-wave potentials, demonstrating that fragmented electrical activity is an independent predictor of early AF recurrence.

5. Limitations

Most of the reviewed studies were observational, retrospective, with a low sample size and event rate, but careful statistical analysis may compensate the mentioned limitations. LVPs were detected using various equipment, commercially available or not, using different averaging and filtering methods. On the other hand, filtered QRS duration was not measured sequentially, considering therapy in all studies, and there was a lack of uniformity of the normality criteria for the diagnosis of LVPs.

False positive LVPs were reported in patients with junctional rhythm with retrograde P-waves, atrial flutter, and incomplete bundle branch block [51–53]. Combined TD and spectral turbulence analysis of the SAECG could improve its predictive value for fatal arrhythmias [54]. The positive predictive accuracy nearly doubled compared to TD or STA, without loss in sensitivity and specificity [54]. A high number of false positive LVPs was reported in myocardial infarction, as well, and in the early postinfarction period; in inferior myocardial infarction in time-domain analysis and anterior myocardial infarction according to STA [54, 55]. Delayed terminal conduction may increase the incidence of false positive results in SAECG, but the incidence of false positive LVPs was significantly lower if the combination of SAECG-QRS, LAS40, and RMS40 was used in patients with incomplete bundle branch block [53]. LVPs detected during sinus rhythm and lost after premature ventricular contractions may be responsible for false positive LVPs, and those revealed by ventricular extrastimuli and concealed during sinus rhythm may cause false negative LVPs [56]. Sensitivity might be low in patients with ventricular tachycardia due to early activation of potential sites of ventricular tachycardia in sinus rhythm, falling within the normal QRS duration [56]. The number of false positive results may be reduced by signal-averaging during premature ventricular stimulation [56].

Larger follow-up studies are needed to confirm the significance and usefulness of LVPs in different cardiac and noncardiac disorders.

6. Conclusions

This chapter brought back into focus SAECG, a noninvasive, low-cost, simple, and rapid method as a predictor of sudden cardiac death, using amplified ECG signals. Even though SAECG is not a routine screening test for sudden cardiac death risk and despite its low positive predictive value for arrhythmic events, LVPs and intra-QRS potentials provide valuable information not only in cardiac but also in extracardiac disorders, including psychiatric disorders, epilepsy, chronic obstructive pulmonary disease, and endocrine disorders. P-wave signal-averaged electrocardiography predicts atrial fibrillation episodes in patients with several disorders, such as hypertension, atrial septal defect, stroke, and chronic obstructive pulmonary disease.

Author details

Ioana Mozos[1]* and Dana Stoian[2]

*Address all correspondence to: ioanamozos@umft.ro

1 Department of Functional Sciences, Victor Babeș University of Medicine and Pharmacy, Timișoara, Romania

2 Department of Internal Medicine, Victor Babeș University of Medicine and Pharmacy, Timișoara, Romania

References

[1] Barbosa PRB, Barbosa EC, Bomfim AS, et al. Clinical assessment of the effect of digital filtering on the detection of ventricular late potentials. Brazilian Journal of Medical and Biological Research. 2002;**35**(11):1285-1292. DOI: 10.1590/S0100-879X2002001100005

[2] Ramos JA, Lopes dos Santos PJ. Parametric modeling in estimating abnormal intra-QRS potentials in signal-averaged electrocardiograms: A subspace identification approach.

In: 16th IFAC Symposium on System Identification, the International Federation of Automatic Control; 11-13 July 2012; Brussels, Belgium, published by Elsevier Ltd.

[3] Abdelghani SA, Rosenthal TM, Morin DP. Surface electrocardiogram predictors of sudden cardiac arrest. Ochsner Journal. 2016;**16**:280-289

[4] Zipes D, Camm J, Borggrefe M, et al. ACC/AHA/ESC 2006 guidelines for management of patients with ventricular arrhythmias and the prevention of sudden cardiac death: A report of the American College of Cardiology/American Heart Association Task Force and the European Society of Cardiology Committee for Practice Guidelines (Writing Committee to develop guidelines for management of patients with ventricular arrhythmias and the prevention of sudden cardiac death). Journal of the American College of Cardiology. 2006;**48**(5):e247-e346. DOI: 10.1016/j.jacc.2006.07.010

[5] Gasparova I, Kubatka P, Opatrilova R, et al. Perspectives and challenges of antioxidant therapy for atrial fibrillation. Naunyn-Schmiedeberg's Archives of Pharmacology. 2017;**390**(1):1-14. DOI: 10.1007/s00210-016-1320-9

[6] Mozoş I, Şerban C, Mihăescu R. Late ventricular potentials in cardiac and extracardiac diseases. In: Breijo-Marquez FR, editor. Cardiac Arrhythmias—New Considerations. InTech; 2012. DOI: 10.5772/25415. Available from: http://www.intechopen.com/books/cardiac-arrhythmias-new-considerations/late-ventricular-potentials-in-cardiac-and-extracardiac-diseases

[7] Goldberger JJ, Cain ME, Hohnloser SH, et al. American Heart Association/American College of Cardiology Foundation/Heart Rhythm Society scientific statement on noninvasive risk stratification techniques for identifying patients at risk for sudden cardiac death. A scientific statement from the American Heart Association Council on Clinical Cardiology Committee on Electrocardiography and Arrhythmias and Council on Epidemiology and Prevention. Journal of the American College of Cardiology. 2008;**52**:1179-1199. DOI: 10.1016/j.hrthm.2008.05.031

[8] Breithardt G, Cain ME, El-Sherif N, et al. Standards for analysis of ventricular late potentials using high-resolution or signal averaged electrocardiography. Journal of the American College of Cardiology. 1991;**17**(5):999-1006. DOI: 10.1161/01.CIR.83.4.1481

[9] Lander P, Berbari EJ, Rajagopalan CV, et al. Critical analysis of the signal-averaged electrocardiogram. Improved identification of late potentials. Circulation. 1993;**87**:105-117. DOI: 10.1161/01.CIR.87.1.105

[10] Askenazi J, Parisi AF, Cohn PF, et al. Value of the QRS complex in assessing left ventricular ejection fraction. American Journal of Cardiology. 1978;**41**(3):491-499

[11] Engel G, Beckerman JG, Froelicher VF, et al. Electrocardiographic arrhythmia risk testing. Current Problems in Cardiology. 2004;**29**:357-432. DOI: 10.1016/j.cpcardiol.2004.02.007

[12] Santangeli P, Infusino F, Sgueglia GA, et al. Ventricular late potentials: A critical overview and current applications. Journal of Electrocardiology. 2008;**41**:318-324. DOI: 10.1016/j.jelectrocard.2008.03.001

[13] Gottfridsson C, Karlsson T, Edvardsson N. The signal-averaged electrocardiogram before and after electrical cardioversion of persistent atrial fibrillation—implications of the sudden change in rhythm. Journal of Electrocardiology. 2011;**44**:242-250. DOI: 10.1016/j.jelectrocard.2010.05.001

[14] Leisy PJ, Coeytaux RR, Wagner GS, et al. ECG-based signal analysis technologies for evaluating patients with acute coronary syndrome: A systematic review. Journal of Electrocardiology. 2013;**46**:92-97. DOI: 10.1016/j.jelectrocard.2012.11.010

[15] Tsiachris D, Silberbauer J, Maccabelli G, et al. Electroanatomical voltage and morphology characteristics in postinfarction patients undergoing ventricular tachycardia ablation pragmatic approach favoring late potentials abolition. Circulation: Arrhythmia and Electrophysiology. 2015;**8**:863-873. DOI: 10.1161/CIRCEP.114.002551

[16] Tahara T, Sogou T, Suezawa C, et al. Filtered QRS duration on signal-averaged electrocardiography correlates with ventricular dyssynchrony assessed by tissue Doppler imaging in patients with reduced ventricular ejection fraction. Journal of Electrocardiology. 2010;**43**:48-53. DOI: 10.1016/j.jelectrocard.2009.06.005

[17] Ohkubo K, Watanabe I, Okumara Y, et al. Analysis of the spatial and transmural dispersion of repolarization and late potentials derived using signal-averaged vector-projected 187-channel high-resolution electrocardiogram in patients with early repolarization pattern. Journal of Arrhythmia. 2014;**30**:446-452. DOI: 10.1016/j.joa.2013.12.002

[18] Lin CY, Chung FP, Lin YJ, et al. Gender differences in patients with arrhythmogenic right ventricular dysplasia/cardiomyopathy: Clinical manifestations, electrophysiological properties, substrate characteristics, and prognosis of radiofrequency catheter ablation. International Journal of Cardiology. 2017;**227**:930-937. DOI: 10.1016/j.ijcard.2016.11.055

[19] Dinov B, Bode K, Koenig S, et al. Signal-averaged electrocardiography as a noninvasive tool for evaluating the outcomes after radiofrequency catheter ablation of ventricular tachycardia in patients with ischemic heart disease: Reassessment of an old tool. Circulation: Arrhythmia and Electrophysiology. 2016;**9**(9). pii: e003673. DOI: 10.1161/CIRCEP.115.003673

[20] Graceffo MA, O'Rourke RA. Cardiac transplant rejection is associated with a decrease in the high-frequency components of the high-resolution, signal averaged electrocardiogram. American Heart Journal. 1996;**132**(4):820-826. DOI: 10.1016/S0002-8703(96)90317-8

[21] Horenstein MS, Idriss SF, Hamilton RM, et al. Efficacy of signal-averaged electrocardiography in the young orthotopic heart transplant patient to detect allograft rejection. Pediatric Cardiology. 2006;**27**:589-593. DOI: 10.1007/s00246-005-1155-5

[22] Mendes VN, Pereira TS, Matos VA. Diagnosis of rejection by analyzing ventricular late potentials in heart transplant patients. Arquivos Brasileiros de Cardiologia. 2016;**106**(2):136-144. DOI: 10.5935/abc.20160011

[23] Rejdak K, Rubaj A, Glowniak A, et al. Analysis of ventricular late potentials in signal-averaged ECG of people with epilepsy. Epilepsia. 2011;**52**(11):2118-2124. DOI: 10.1111/j.1528-1167.2011.03270.x

[24] Mozos I. Ventricular arrhythmia risk in noncardiac diseases. In: Aronow WS, editor. Cardiac Arrhythmias—Mechanisms, Pathophysiology, and Treatment. InTech; 2014. DOI: 10.5772/57164. Available from: http://www.intechopen.com/books/cardiac-arrhythmias-mechanisms-pathophysiology-and-treatment/ventricular-arrhythmia-risk-in-noncardiac-diseases

[25] Mozos I. Arrhythmia risk and obesity. Journal of Molecular and Genetic Medicine. 2014: S1. DOI: 10.4172/1747-0862.S1-006

[26] Mozos I. Laboratory markers of ventricular arrhythmia risk in renal failure. BioMed Research International. 509204. DOI: 10.1155/2014/509204. [Epub: May 26, 2014]

[27] Buzea CA, Dan GA, Dan AR, et al. Role of signal-averaged electrocardiography and ventricular late potentials in patients with chronic obstructive pulmonary disease. Romanian Journal of Internal Medicine. 2015;**53**(2):133-139. DOI: 10.1515/rjim-2015-0018

[28] Antoniou CK, Bournellis I, Papadopoulos A, et al. Prevalence of late potentials on signal-averaged ECG in patients with psychiatric disorders. International Journal of Cardiology. 2016;**222**:557-561. DOI: 10.1016/j.ijcard.2016.07.270

[29] Bivanco-Lima D, Souza Santos Id, Vannucchi AM, et al. Cardiovascular risk in individuals with depression. Revista da Associação Médica Brasileira. 1992;**59**(3):298-304. DOI: 10.1016/j.ramb.2012.12.006

[30] Biet M, Morin N, Lessard-Beaudoin M, et al. Prolongation of action potential duration and QT interval during epilepsy linked to increased contribution of neuronal sodium channels to cardiac late Na^+ current: Potential mechanism for sudden death in epilepsy. Circulation: Arrhythmia and Electrophysiology. 2015;**8**(4):912-920. DOI: 10.1161/CIRCEP.114.002693

[31] Svalheim S, Aurlien D, Amlie JP, et al. Signal-averaged and standard electrocardiography in patients with newly diagnosed epilepsy. Epilepsy & Behavior. 2012;**25**(4):543-545. DOI: 10.1016/j.yebeh.2012.09.023

[32] Carjea MI. Prevalence of late ventricular potentials in patients with chronic obstructive lung disease. Pneumologia. 2003;**52**(3-4):181-183

[33] Yildiz P, Tükek T, Akkaya V, et al. Ventricular arrhythmias in patients with COPD are associated with QT dispersion. Chest. 2002;**122**(6):2055-2061. DOI: 10.1378/chest.122.6.2055

[34] Maffei P, Martini C, Milanesi A, et al. Late potentials and ventricular arrhythmias in acromegaly. International Journal of Cardiology. 2005;**104**(2):197-203. DOI: 10.1016/j.ijcard.2004.12.010

[35] Mosca S, Paolillo S, Colao A, et al. Cardiovascular involvement in patients affected by acromegaly: An appraisal. International Journal of Cardiology. 2013;**167**:1712-1718. DOI: 10.1016/j.ijcard.2012.11.109

[36] Herrmann BL, Bruch C, Saller B, et al. Occurrence of ventricular late potentials in patients with active acromegaly. Clinical Endocrinology (Oxford). 2001;**55**(2):201-207. DOI: 10.1046/j.1365-2265.2001.01319.x

[37] Ker J. Thyroxine and cardiac electrophysiology—a forgotten physiological duo? Thyroid Research. 2012;**5**(1):8. DOI: 10.1186/1756-6614-5-8

[38] Schippinger W, Buchinger W, Schubert B, et al. Late potentials in high resolution ECG in thyroid gland dysfunction. Acta Medica Austriaca. 1995;**22**(4):73-74

[39] Kamenicky P, Redheuil A, Roux C, et al. Cardiac structure and function in Cushing's syndrome: A cardiac magnetic resonance imaging study. Journal of Clinical Endocrinology and Metabolism. 2014;**99**(11):E2144-E2153. DOI: 10.1210/jc.2014-1783

[40] Lin CC. Analysis of unpredictable intra-QRS potentials in signal-averaged electrocardiograms using an autoregressive moving average prediction model. Medical Engineering & Physics. 2010;**32**(2):136-144. DOI: 10.1016/j.medengphy.2009.11.001

[41] Lin CC. Analysis of abnormal intra-QRS potentials in signal-averaged electrocardiograms using a radial basis function neural network. Sensors. 2016;**16**(10):1580. DOI: 10.3390/s16101580

[42] Barbosa PRB, de Souza Bomfim A, Barbosa EC, et al. Spectral turbulence analysis of the signal-averaged electrocardiogram of the atrial activation as predictor of recurrence of idiopathic and persistent atrial fibrillation. International Journal of Cardiology. 2006;**107**:307-316. DOI: 10.1016/j.ijcard.2005.03.073

[43] Buzea CA, Dan AR, Delcea C, et al. P wave signal-averaged electrocardiography in patients with chronic obstructive pulmonary disease. Romanian Journal of Internal Medicine. 2015;**53**(4):315-320. DOI: 10.1515/rjim-2015-0040

[44] Yogodawa K, Seino Y, Ohara T, et al. Prediction of atrial fibrillation after ischemic stroke using P-wave signal averaged electrocardiography. Journal of Cardiology. 2013;**61**:49-52. DOI: 10.1016/j.jjcc.2012.08.013

[45] Aytemir K, Amasyali B, Abali G, et al. The signal-averaged P-wave duration is longer in hypertensive patients with history of paroxysmal atrial fibrillation as compared to those without. International Journal of Cardiology. 2005;**103**:37-40. DOI: 10.1016/j.ijcard.2004.08.027

[46] Budeus M, Hennersdorf M, Röhlen S, et al. Prediction of atrial fibrillation after coronary artery bypass grafting: The role of chemoreflex sensitivity and P wave signal averaged ECG. International Journal of Cardiology. 2006;**106**:67-74. DOI: 10.1016/j.ijcard.2004.12.062

[47] Thilen U, Carlson J, Platonov PG, et al. Atrial myocardial pathoelectrophysiology in adults with a secundum atrial septal defect is unaffected by closure of the defect. A study using high resolution signal-averaged orthogonal P-wave technique. International Journal of Cardiology. 2009;**132**:364-368. DOI: 10.1016/j.ijcard.2007.11.101

[48] Auriti A, Aspromonte N, Ceci V, et al. Signal-averaged P-wave in hypertension for the risk of paroxysmal atrial fibrillation. Pacing and Clinical Electrophysiology. 1995;**18**(Part II):1096

[49] Darbar D, Hardy A, Haines JL, et al. Prolonged signal-averaged P-wave duration as an intermediate phenotype for familial atrial fibrillation. Journal of the American College of Cardiology. 2008;**51**(11):1083-1089. DOI: 10.1016/j.jacc.2007.11.058

[50] Dakos G, Konstantinou D, Chatzizisis YS, et al. P wave analysis with wavelets identifies hypertensive patients at risk of recurrence of atrial fibrillation: A case-control study and 1 year follow-up. Journal of Electrocardiology. 2015;**48**:845-852. DOI: 10.1016/j.jelectrocard.2015.07.012

[51] Schrem SS, Nachamie M, Weiss E. False positive signal-averaged electrocardiogram produced by atrial flutter. American Heart Journal. 1990;**120**(3):698-699. DOI: 10.1016/0002-8703(90)90033-T

[52] Taylor E, Effron M, Veltri EP. False positive signal-averaged ECG produced by junctional rhythm with retrograde P waves. American Heart Journal. 1992;**123**(6):1701-1703

[53] Manolis AS, Chiladakis JA, Malakos JS, et al. Abnormal signal-averaged electrocardiograms in patients with incomplete right bundle-branch block. Clinical Cardiology. 1997;**20**(1):17-22. DOI: 10.1002/clc.4960200106

[54] Vazquez R, Caref EB, Torres F, et al. Improved diagnostic value of combined time and frequency domain analysis of the signal-averaged electrocardiogram after myocardial infarction. Journal of the American College of Cardiology. 1999;**33**:385-394. DOI: 10.1016/S0735-1097(98)00581-6

[55] El-Sherif N, Ursell SN, Bekheit S, et al. Prognostic significance of the signal-averaged electrocardiogram depends on the time of recording in the post-infarction period. American Heart Journal. 1989;**118**:256-264

[56] Ho DS, Daly M, Richards DAB, et al. Behavior of late potentials on the body surface during programmed ventricular stimulation. Journal of the American College of Cardiology. 1996;**28**:1283-1291. DOI: 10.1016/S0735-1097(96)00297-5.

Chapter 4

Non-invasive Detection and Compression of Fetal Electrocardiogram

Xin Gao

Additional information is available at the end of the chapter

http://dx.doi.org/10.5772/intechopen.69920

Abstract

Noninvasive detection of fetal electrocardiogram (FECG) from abdominal ECG recordings is highly dependent on typical statistical signal processing techniques such as independent component analysis (ICA), adaptive noise filtering, and multichannel blind deconvolution. In contrast to the previous multichannel FECG extraction methods, several recent schemes for single-channel FECG extraction such as the extended Kalman filter (EKF), extended Kalman smoother (EKS), template subtraction (TS), and support vector regression (SVR) for detecting *R* waves on ECG, are evaluated via the quantitative metrics such as sensitivity (SE), positive predictive value (PPV), *F*-score, detection error rate (DER), and range of accuracy. A correlation predictor that combines with multivariable gray model (GM) is also proposed for sequential ECG data compression, which displays better percent root mean-square difference (PRD) than those of Sabah's scheme for fixed and predicted compression ratio (CR). Automatic calculation on fetal heart rate (FHR) on the reconstructed FECG from mixed signals of abdominal ECG recordings is also experimented with sample synthetic ECG data. Sample data on FHR and T/QRS for both physiological case and pathological case are simulated in a 10-min time sequence.

Keywords: noninvasive detection, FECG, FHR, gray prediction, data compression

1. Introduction

Fetal electrocardiogram (FECG) and fetal heart rate (FHR) represent crucial indices for clinical examination and medical diagnosis during pregnancy [1–7, 9–11, 20, 31–36]. In the past decades, multiple systems dynamically monitoring FECG [5, 6, 15, 19, 20, 25–27, 29–31, 35] had been designed for the use of prenatal diagnosis in fetal heart disease, real-time surveillance during both natural and cesarean delivery, as well as the antenatal and intrapartum assessment. Due to the large amount of FECG data for processing in successive monitoring time, enormous storage equipment with durable maintenance is necessary in the design of practical devices [8]: for instance, the double-channel Holter system requires a memory of 82 megabits for sampled data storage with the resolution of 11 bits and 360 Hz for sampling rate per channel every day. Hence, the design of dynamic system urges solutions for better improvements in practical use for noninvasive FECG detection and compression in portable devices and sensing utilities. A variety of typical FECG extraction techniques [2–5, 9, 14–17, 19, 20, 23–26, 35, 36] had been established for both theoretical study and subsequent practical hardware design [18, 25, 29]. A few classical compression methods [13] introduced for efficient data restoration include polynomial fitting, predictive coding, and orthogonal transform-domain compression, where the principle of data compression is to minimize redundancy at comparatively low penalty of distortion and losing useful information [8]. The correlative models exploiting the correlation information between adjacent QRS waves for sequential prediction suggest an efficient scheme for FECG data compression [8].

The classical schemes for noninvasive FECG extraction over the past 30 years mainly comprise of adaptive signal processing with noise cancellation, spatial filtering techniques, and singular-value decomposition (SVD), to name a few [19, 25]; while the major shortcomings of these schemes were high sensitivity of fetal location and maternal movements, difficulties in extracting P/T waves, and incomplete capture of ECG diagrams [19, 35, 36]. In statistical signal processing, independent component analysis (ICA) [10, 16] aims at computationally separating a mixed signal (with multivariate components) into non-Gaussian signals, where the decomposed signals are assumed to be statistically independent within each other. A variety of methods have been developed for noninvasive FECG extraction since the ICA technique was applied in this research field such as the fourth-order cumulant-based scheme with diagonal approximation proposed by Lathauwer et al. [16], the Joint Approximate Diagonalization of Eigen-matrices (JADE) scheme by Zarzoso [34], Hyvarinen's fast invariant-point method with the ICA principle [10], and the wavelet transform-based infomax algorithm by Jafari and Chambers [12]. Theoretical study on noninvasive FECG extraction methods also employed the ICA-based JADE method with high-order blind identification, the joint detection schemes such as the JADE algorithm with multiple unknown signal extraction, multichannel blind deconvolution [37], and applying the sparse representation of FECG components derived from ICA in the compressed domain [21]. While some previous techniques for noninvasive FECG detection had been considerably mature enough, the challenging issues [4, 28] that have been recognized consist of saving computational cost in abdominal ECG recordings, performing efficient restoration on ECG data, and realizing the practical design (as oriented for low cost, low power, and high integration [29]) for portable FECG monitoring systems. As a result, meeting the balance of recent technical advances with the experimental design on practical systems for noninvasive FECG data-processing devices becomes a crucial task within our investigation.

In this chapter, we present a general study on several categories of algorithms in the field of noninvasive FECG detection, and carry out a performance analysis via several metrics on the state-of-the-art schemes for extracting FECG using sample databases [2, 19, 21]. We proposed a unified approach for the dynamic system design on FECG detection, with a block diagram on noninvasive ECG extraction by collaborating data-processing techniques on weak signal detection and parameter estimation [8]. Utilizing the correlations between adjacent QRS waves of mixed FECG and maternal ECG (MECG), we derived an improved scheme for ECG compression by predicting minimum mean-square error (MMSE), performing integer wavelet transform, quantization, run-length coding, and arithmetic coding for better realization of FECG data compression [8]. Considerably high compression ratio (CR) with feasible lower distortion in contrast to Sabah's scheme is achieved in condition of preserving the most useful message in the compressed FECG data sequence. Simulations rely on the GM(1, 1) model for gray prediction on CR and percent root mean-square difference (PRD) [8]. We also use the sample synthetic ECG data to fulfill the task of automatic estimation on fetal heart rate (FHR) from the reconstructed FECG.

2. Methodology

The waveform of ECG as depicted in **Figure 1** comprises *P*, *T* waves, and the central QRS interval in a regular period of time [8, 24]. Since continuous ECG monitoring explicitly indicates the exposure of regular heart rate, heartbeat rate with amplitude and duration, prior information on the symptoms of potential heart disease is the most important data reference on medical diagnosis. FECG represents weak signals containing a few strong interferences such as MECG with baseline wander, power line interference and additive noise, while the

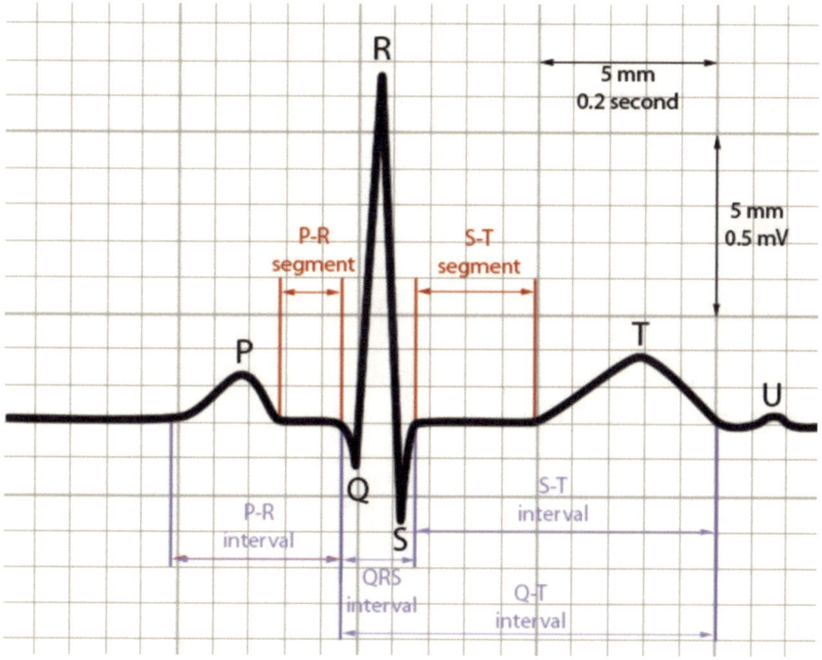

Figure 1. A diagram on the waveform of ECG in a normal period.

noninvasive techniques aim to eliminate these strong disturbances by directly or indirectly measuring FECG via a few properly located electrodes on the maternal abdomen during pregnancy.

Previous schemes such as fetal scalp electrode monitoring, belong to the category of invasive FECG detection (by either scalp electrode or vaginal ultrasound). However, the invasive schemes have obvious shortcomings such as causing pains and injury to the maternal body, and inducing potential risks on uterus infection to the developing fetus. The fetal ECG detection schemes discussed in this chapter belong to noninvasive techniques, indicating no damage or penetration through maternal or fetal skins.

In general cases on noninvasive detection, the mixed ECG was acquired by multiple electrodes in different locations from both thoracic and abdominal regions on a pregnant woman. For instance, the common diagnostic tool for noninvasive ECG recordings usually adopts 8-lead or 12-lead electrode placement (with symmetric electrodes) [2, 20, 41], which had been derived via clinical validation in a couple of periods. The FECG components in multi-lead abdominal recordings are mutually dependent with each other on the fetal position and the electrical conduction toward the maternal abdominal skin. Due to the variations of each component, calculating linear combinations of multichannel outputs generally enhance the signal-to-noise ratio (SNR) of FECG [20]. Meanwhile, since the main electrical axis of the fetal heart position is *a priori* uncertain, in order to increase the possibilities that the calculated nonphysiological leads contain significant FECG components, it is often chosen to compute a set of four linear combinations for equal weights, that is, the position angles correspond with 0°, 45°, 90°, and 135° for the 8-lead placement [2, 20]. Similarly, a 12-lead ECG placement (12 leads calculated using 10 electrodes, in which 6 chest electrodes provide information on the heart's horizontal plane and 4 limb electrodes on the heart's vertical plane) illustrates a more cohesive diagram on the accurate electrical activity of the heart by recording information through 12 different perspectives, where the instruction with specific details on the 12-lead placement guide was illustrated in Ref. [41]. **Figure 2(a)** and **(b)** illustrate the typical 8-lead electrode placement [2, 20] for noninvasive FECG detection and 12-lead electrode replacement [41] for ECG monitoring, respectively.

Among the representative FECG extraction schemes as mentioned above, while blind source separation (BSS) through ICA [16] was previously regarded as having achieved considerably satisfactory results, the demands for multiple signal inputs (typically 8 channels), in addition to the pre-assumption of linearity between MECG and maternal component in the abdominal ECG recordings and monitoring, were put forward as setbacks toward real-time needs in practical implementations [19]. While simulations on the actual relationship between MECG and maternal component in the abdominal ECG were recorded as single-channel inputs, a few other nonlinear schemes proposed recently can be enumerated as given below: the Bayesian filtering framework using the modified dynamic models via several model-based filters such as the extended Kalman filter (EKF), extended Kalman smoother (EKS), unscented Kalman filter (UKF), and wavelet denoising for synthetic ECG data [22, 26]; the ANFIS system [4], in contrast to normalized least mean squares and polynomial networks, for the identification and extraction of FECG from the aligned MECG; the cascaded framework of EKF (for MECG estimation) with ANFIS (for FECG extraction) on both synthetic and actual ECG data in

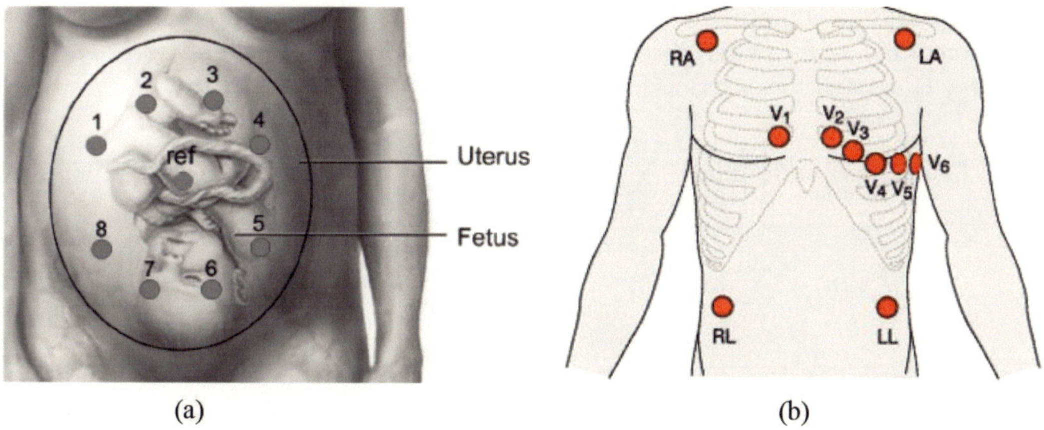

Figure 2. The illustrations of electrodes on: (a) configuration of 8-lead placement for fetal ECG detection; (b) configuration of 12-lead placement for ECG monitoring: the 6 chest electrodes V_1–V_6 show the locations on precordial placements, the 4 limb electrodes show the locations on extremity placements (RA–right arm, LA–left arm, RL–right leg, LL–left leg).

contrast to single EKF, EKS [3], template adaptation (TA) [2], nonparametric detection scheme, and modified template subtraction on sequential data processing [19]; the singular spectrum analysis-based fetal heart signal extraction [9], the fetal heartbeat detection algorithm by the integration of Hilbert transform and nonlinear state-space projections [36], and by supporting vector regression [35]; and a few other clinically adopted noninvasive FECG detection methods from multilead abdominal ECG recordings, see Refs. [4, 5, 15, 17, 20, 33], and the references therein.

For nonstationary signals such as ECG, classical evaluation criteria such as the MMSE principle and predictive coding may generate considerably large prediction errors especially when the amplitude of signal depicts quick fluctuation [8]. Consider two adjacent QRS waveforms with strong relativity in successive phases, let $x(n)$ and $y(n)$ be the input and output of ECG signals, respectively; we observe a sequential data of p points of the former QRS waveform in order to predict the present waveform at the minor cost of generating prediction errors. The predictor output is expressed as [8]:

$$y(n) = \sum_{i=1}^{p} \alpha_i x(n-i-T) \quad (1)$$

where α_i denotes the coefficients of system cascades which can be obtained by Yule-Walker equations and T stands for the average time period between the intervals of R waves.

The prediction error $\varepsilon(n)$ can be calculated via [8]

$$\varepsilon(n) = x(n) - y(n) = x(n) - \sum_{i=1}^{p} \alpha_i x(n-i-T) \quad (2)$$

where a set of consecutive p points represents the orders of correlation predictor.

Since the prediction is processed between two adjacent QRS waveforms, let us denote such kind of prediction as the twin-*R* correlative prediction [8]. In mean-square scales, we express the energy E_p of prediction errors as [8]

$$\begin{aligned} E_p = E[\varepsilon^2(n)] &= E\left\{\left[x(n) - \sum_{i=1}^{p} \alpha_i x(n-i-T)\right]^2\right\} \\ &= E\left\{x^2(n) - 2\sum_{i=1}^{p} \alpha_i x(n) x(n-i-T) + \sum_{i=1}^{p} \alpha_i \sum_{j=1}^{p} \alpha_j x(n-i-T) x(n-j-T)\right\} \\ &= R(0) - 2\sum_{i=1}^{p} \alpha_i R(i+T) + \sum_{i=1}^{p} \alpha_i \sum_{j=1}^{p} \alpha_j R(j-i) \end{aligned} \tag{3}$$

The correlation coefficients of input ECG waves can be calculated via [8]

$$R(m) = \frac{1}{N} \sum_{n=1}^{N-1} x(n) x(n-m) \tag{4}$$

Simplifying Eq. (4) by taking $\frac{\partial E_p}{\partial \alpha_i} = 0$ to obtain a minimum for E_p ($m = 0, 1, \ldots, p-1$) yields [8]

$$\sum_{i=1}^{p-1} \alpha_i R(m-i) = R(m+T), \qquad i = 0, 1, \ldots, p\text{–}1 \tag{5}$$

Constructing the matrix of correlation coefficients by combining Eqs. (3)–(5) yields the linear algebraic equations as follows [8]

$$\begin{bmatrix} R(0) & R(1) & \cdots & R(p-1) \\ R(1) & R(0) & \cdots & R(p-2) \\ \vdots & \vdots & \ddots & \vdots \\ R(p-1) & R(p-2) & \cdots & R(0) \end{bmatrix} \begin{bmatrix} \alpha_0 \\ \alpha_1 \\ \vdots \\ \alpha_{p-1} \end{bmatrix} = \begin{bmatrix} R(T) \\ R(T+1) \\ \vdots \\ R(T+p-1) \end{bmatrix} \tag{6}$$

Solving the equation group in Eq. (6) as above yields the numerical coefficients of each α_i.

The lifting wavelet transform (LWT) has been recognized as a strong implementation when combined with a few algorithms such as integer square zero-tree wavelet coding [8]. Splitting, predicting, and updating symbols, are three steps in the lifting scheme of a typical LWT. The proposed scheme is presented as follows: the first step is to split the ECG data sequence $\{e_j\}$ into two sequences $\{o_{j\text{-}1}\}$ and $\{e_{j\text{-}1}\}$ that stands for odd and even numerals via [8]

$$\text{split } (e_j) = (e_{j-1}, o_{j-1}) \tag{7}$$

Second, with respect to the predictor filter group *P* and the earlier even sequence $\{e_{j\text{-}1}\}$, the odd sequence $\{o_{j\text{-}1}\}$ is predicted by exploiting correlativity information such as [8]

$$o_{j-1} := o_{j-1} - P(e_{j-1}) \tag{8}$$

The last step of updating claims that some integral characteristics as those of integrity for the original $\{e_j\}$ need to be preserved for constructing a better subset $\{e_{j-1}\}$. As a result, we adopt an updating filter U that exploits the discrepancy between a specific parameter (i.e., mean, variance, or wavelet vanishing moments) and $\{e_j\}$, where this step is proceeded by [8]

$$e_{j-1} := e_{j-1} + U(o_{j-1}) \tag{9}$$

The inverse transform of LWT for signal reconstruction can be similarly expressed via [8]

$$\begin{cases} e_{j-1} := e_{j-1} - U(o_{j-1}) \\ o_{j-1} := o_{j-1} + P(e_{j-1}) \\ e_j = \text{Merge}\,(e_{j-1}, o_{j-1}) \end{cases} \tag{10}$$

The iteration procedures as performed in Ref. [8], applied a (4, 2) LWT for the decomposition and reconstruction of ECG signals, which can be proceeded by [8]

$$\begin{cases} o_j[n] := e_{j-1}[n] + \left\lfloor \frac{1}{16}\{(e_{j-1}[n+2]) - 9(e_{j-1}[n+2]) + e_{j-1}[n-1]) + e_{j-1}[n-1]\} + \frac{1}{2} \right\rfloor \\ e_j[n] := e_{j-1}[n] + \left\lfloor \frac{1}{4}(o_j[n] + o_j[n-1]) + \frac{1}{2} \right\rfloor \end{cases} \tag{11}$$

where $\lfloor . \rfloor$ denotes the execution of the round-off operation.

The advantages of LWT compared to other wavelet transform methods are displayed in the following scenarios [8]: (i) less dependence for the down-sampling of low pass and high pass signal components and easier realization on the inverse operation of LWT; (ii) reduced execution times by avoiding calculating floating points coming from the integer coefficients; (iii) the implementation of hardware circuits is also much easier; and (iv) guaranteed quality for signal recovery free of boundary continuation in any type.

The procedure of our proposed twin-R correlation predictor for improving sequential ECG compression is presented as below [8]: let us denote the implement D as the first-order time delay and P_i as the location of the ith R-wave; $\mathbf{A}_j = \{\alpha_{j,0}, \alpha_{j,1}, \ldots, \alpha_{j,p\text{-}1}\}$ stands for the aggregated coefficients for the twin-R interval of the jth ECG sequence. We take the following steps to perform this task:

Step 1. For the original ECG signal with length N, initially perform the first-order prediction to reduce the DC components of the signals; let $z(n)$ be the redundancy within smooth district of the ECG samples calling for elimination, the residual term $z(n)$ is now expressed as

$$z(n) = x(n) - x(n-1), \qquad n = 0, 1, \ldots, N-1. \tag{12}$$

Step 2. While P_i, the locations of R-wave for each QRS waveform, have been identified, compute each T_i by deducing $T_i = P_{i+1} - P_i$, and estimate the central position of the adjacent twin-R

waves, where $m_i = (P_{i+1} + P_i)/2$. This step speeds up higher recognition rate and operation time, and bears negative effects such as noise interference or baseline shift.

Step 3. Perform the correlation prediction for $z(n)$ similar to Eq. (2):

$$d(n) = z(n) - \sum_{k=0}^{p-1} \alpha_{j,k} z(n-i-T_{i-1}), m_i - l \leq m_i + l, l = \min(m_{i-1} - m_{i-2}, m_i - m_{i-1})/2, i = 1, \ldots, N_j. \tag{13}$$

where $d(n)$ denotes the signal of prediction error, p and N_j stand for the order of predictor and the R-wave counts of the jth ECG data sequence, respectively. Without loss of generality, we adopt $p = 4$. The kth prediction coefficient $\alpha_{j,k}$ of each compressed 16-bit ECG sequence was obtained via the splitting process in Step 1. Due to the slow drift for the QRS waveform, an interval of 30 seconds was used to partition this data stream. Note that we implemented the same predictors for continuous QRS waveforms of the same ECG data in order to reduce computational cost and enhance the efficiency for ECG data compression.

Step 4. Update the (4, 2) LWT on the signal $d(n)$ via Eq. (12), where the length of $w(n)$ is preserved as N. For the subband signal $w(n)$ containing $\{o_i(n) = 1,2,3,4\}$ and the approximated signal $e_4(n)$, their length are constructed as $N/2$, $N/4$, $N/8$, $N/16$, and $N/16$, respectively.

Step 5. Perform scalar quantization, run-length coding, and arithmetic coding for $w(n)$. While a few zero-coefficients appear after quantization toward $w(n)$, these successive zeros can be removed via run-length searching so as to shorten the ECG data sequence. Variable quantization coefficients are selected in this procedure; after run-length coding each ECG data sequence is merged by three parts: the constructed bit streams, vector P_i for R-wave localization, and the twin-R predictor coefficients $\mathbf{A}_j = \{\alpha_{j,0}, \alpha_{j,1}, \ldots, \alpha_{j,p\text{-}1}\}$.

The flowchart of this scheme as described above is depicted in the block diagram of **Figure 3**, where the prediction step is associated with the compressed ECG data stream.

Since the proposed scheme is invertible for decompression, we need to observe the correlativity and fluctuation tendency between two sequential ECG data; hence, a Lemma is presented for the derivation of ECG data prediction via the single-variable gray model [8].

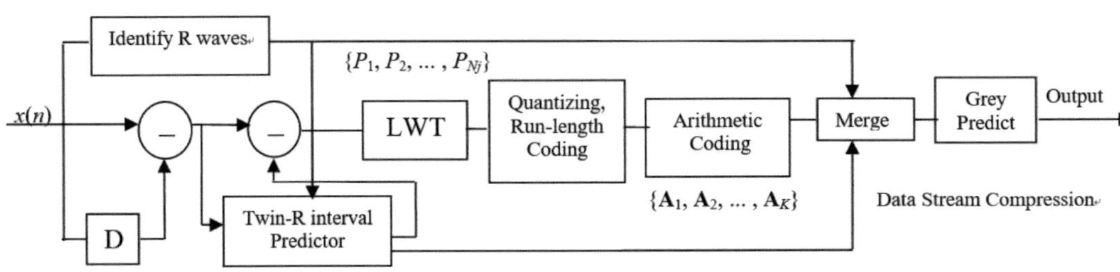

Figure 3. The block diagram of unified twin-*R* predictive method for ECG sequential data compression.

Lemma 1 [8]: Consider a stationary sequence $T_0 = \{T_0(k) \mid k = 1,\dots, n\} = \{T_0(1),\dots, T_0(n)\}$, where k represents the time point. Let us observe a number of m sequences as reference where $T_i = \{T_i(k) \mid k = 1, 2,\dots, n\} = \{T_i(1), T_i(2),\dots, T_i(n)\}$, $i = 1, 2,\dots, n$. Define ξ_k as the correlation coefficient of the kth reference sequence with respect to the starting sequence T_0 at time k,

$$\xi_k = \frac{\min_i \min_k |T_0(k) - T_i(k)| + \rho \max_i \max_k |T_0(k) - T_i(k)|}{|T_0(k) - T_i(k)| + \rho \max_i \max_k |T_0(k) - T_i(k)|} \tag{14}$$

where $\rho \in [0,1)$ denotes the resolution coefficient (and without loss of generality it is often taking expectation of $\rho = 0.5$), $\min_i \min_k |T_0(k) - T_i(k)|$ and $\max_i \max_i |T_i(k) - T_0(k)|$ represents the minimum and maximum difference value between two-levels, respectively. In the gray system theory, $r_i = \frac{1}{n}\sum_{k=1}^{n} \xi_k$ denotes the relevance of sequence T_i to T_0. Geometric similarity on two sequences reflects the degree of correlativity.

Consider the ith sequence $T_i = \{T_i(1), T_i(2),\dots, T_i(n)\}$, the initialized sequence of original T_i is written as $\overline{T} = (1, T(2)/T(1), \dots T(n)/T(1))$, and the correlation factor σ_i can be computed via $\sigma_i = \sum_{k=1}^{N} kT_i(k) - \sum_{k=1}^{N} T_i(k) \sum_{k=1}^{N} \frac{k}{n}$, which has the possibility of being either positive or negative. For instance, in the simplest case of $i = 1, 2$, the sequential expression of T_i is formulated as [8]

$$T_i = \left(1, \frac{T_i(1)}{T_i(2)}, \frac{T_i(1)}{T_i(3)}, \dots, \frac{T_i(1)}{T_i(k)}\right), i = 1, 2; k = N \tag{15}$$

According to Lemma 1, the degree of correlativity is measured by solving Eq. (14). Note that if $\text{sign}(\sigma_1/\sigma_n)\text{sign}(\sigma_2/\sigma_n) = 1$, a positive relevance is justified between T_1 and T_2; conversely, a negative relevance is justified when $\text{sign}(\sigma_1/\sigma_n)\text{sign}(\sigma_2/\sigma_n) = -1$. In more general cases such as ECG data sequence, the correlation factor σ_n can be approximately estimated via [8]

$$\sigma_n = \sum_{k=1}^{n} k^2 - \left(\sum_{k=1}^{n} k^2\right) \Big/ n \tag{16}$$

In the gray system theory, the single variable GM(1, 1) model is often applied to predict the upcoming sequence number and estimate the missed numerical values between time intervals, for the processing of ECG data, we just equalize the corresponding parameters in the time domain, and deduce the gray predictor in the scenario as follows:

The least square (LS) update consists of a whitening procedure through constructing a differential equation in the whitening process with its estimate, and a discretization process for the residuals, which is formulated as [8]:

$$\frac{dT_i^{(1)}}{dt} + aT_i^{(1)} = u, \hat{a} = (a, u)^T \tag{17}$$

$$\hat{\mathbf{a}} = (\mathbf{B}_i^T \mathbf{B}_i)^{-1} \mathbf{B}_i^T \mathbf{Y}_1 \tag{18}$$

$$\mathbf{B}_i = \begin{bmatrix} -\frac{1}{2}(T_i^{(1)}(1) + T_i^{(1)}(2)) & 1 \\ -\frac{1}{2}(T_i^{(1)}(2) + T_i^{(1)}(3)) & 1 \\ \vdots & \vdots \\ -\frac{1}{2}(T_i^{(1)}(n-1) + T_i^{(1)}(n)) & 1 \end{bmatrix}, \mathbf{Y}_i = \begin{bmatrix} T_i^{(1)}(2) \\ T_i^{(1)}(3) \\ \vdots \\ T_i^{(1)}(n) \end{bmatrix} \tag{19}$$

where $\mathbf{B}_i$ and $\mathbf{Y}_i$ denote the data matrix and data vector of GM(1, 1) model, respectively.

A general solution to the matrix equations above is given by [8]

$$T_i^{(1)}(k+1) = \left(T_i^{(0)}(1) - \frac{u}{a}\right)e^{ak} + \frac{u}{a} \tag{20}$$

Determining the model parameters (a, u) yields the past or upcoming numerical values from this predictive GM(1, 1) model. Note that the constructed gray model indicates coincidence with the time-variant extrapolate prediction. In harsh conditions, due to the scarcity of prior information and ambiguity of system on ECG data processing, this predictive GM model is useful since only four adjacent continuous data points are needed from the least data sample.

Because the quality of FECG reflects crucial information on fetal heart rate (FHR) and its beat-to-beat variability [9], the cascaded system design for noninvasive FECG extraction may often involve a post-processing stage such as adaptive noise cancellation or wavelet denoising [12, 22, 34]. FHR is usually estimated via the ratio of 60 to the average time period (s) on a sequence of adjacent intervals from R waves, while estimating FHR technically requires shaping fetal QRS complexes by capturing data via multichannel maternal abdominal ECG recordings [2, 15, 19–21, 23, 26, 30, 32], and by adopting a few other sensing technologies through the Doppler ultrasound devices [37], fetal phonocardiography [1], as well as superconducting magneto-cardiography [33]. Wearable devices on ECG rhythm recording via potential mapping on the wrist/arm surface skin [42] also urge collaborative concerns from industry field toward our theoretically proposed algorithmic study.

3. Performance metrics

The diagnostic tests in biomedical engineering often employ a set of performance metrics in order to evaluate the validity of tests in the subjects on study. In ECG detection, the parameters of true positive (TP), false negative (FN), and false positive (FP) are called from the counts of detected R-peaks. We denote TP as the number of correctly detected R peaks, FN stands for the number of missed R peaks, and FP represents the number of noise spikes detected as R peaks. Hence, the measures of sensitivity (SE) and positive predictive values (PPV) are formulated as [19, 30]:

$$SE = \frac{TP}{TP + FN} \times 100\% \tag{21}$$

$$PPV = \frac{TP}{TP + FP} \times 100\% \tag{22}$$

The F-score, known as the harmonic mean of SE and PPV, is expressed as [2, 21]:

$$F\text{–}score = 2 \cdot \frac{SE \times PPV}{SE + PPV} = \frac{2 \times TP}{2 \times TP + FP + FN} \tag{23}$$

Since the total number of R-wave peaks is the sum of TP, FN, and FP, the detection error rate (DER) is now denoted as [30]:

$$DER = \frac{FP + FN}{TP + FP + FN} \times 100\% \tag{24}$$

For each DER, the metric of accuracy = 1 – DER yields the same expression as defined in Ref. [19].

The percent root mean-square difference (PRD) represents a fidelity measure for some data compression scheme on the reconstructed/predicted signal in contrast to the original ECG, where the PRD value is numerically calculated as follows [13]:

$$PRD = \frac{\sqrt{\sum_{n=1}^{p} [x(n) - y(n)]^2}}{\sum_{n=1}^{p} x^2(n)} \times 100 \tag{25}$$

where $x(n)$ and $y(n)$ correspondingly represent samples of the original and the reconstructed/predicted ECG data sequences and the length of sequence is p.

Regarding the compression ratio (CR) defined as the proportion of uncompressed size to compressed size for a finite data sequence, or the ratio of uncompressed data rate to compressed data rate for streaming media signals of infinite size such as video or audio [38], for each compression scheme, there is a PRD value corresponding to a required CR.

For synthetic ECG data, consider the abdominal ECG $w(n)$ in case of a single-channel dynamic model, which is nonlinearly synthesized via the MECG $m(n)$, FECG $f(n)$, and the additive white noise $\eta(n)$, and hence, the composite signal is modeled as [19]:

$$w(n) = \hat{m}(n) + \hat{f}(n) = \hat{m}(n) + f(n) + \eta(n) \tag{26}$$

where $\hat{m}(n)$ and $\hat{f}(n)$ denote the nonlinear expressions of MECG and FECG, respectively. Since the noise power in $\eta(n)$ can be adjusted to test the performance of each noninvasive FECG detection scheme [19, 30], for some ECG data sequence with a length of p periodical R peaks, the fetal to maternal signal-to-noise ratio (fmSNR) can be calculated via [19]:

$$fmSNR = 10\log_{10}\left(\frac{\sum_{n=1}^{p}[\hat{f}(n)]^2}{\sum_{n=1}^{p}[\hat{m}(n)]^2}\right) \tag{27}$$

Up till now, we have presented a concise study for the keynote noninvasive techniques and quantitative metrics on FECG detection, with an emphasis on single-channel FECG extraction via nonlinear dynamic models. We proposed a flowchart of processing ECG data sequence by means of LWT and the unified twin-*R* correlation predictor by implementing GM(1,1) model for ECG data compression.

In the next section, we will present three sets of experiments for the qualitative and quantitative evaluation on several noninvasive FECG detection schemes [2, 19, 21], the proposed twin-*R* correlative ECG compression scheme via a widely used ECG database [8], and automatic FHR estimation over a sample sequence of synthetic ECG data [40].

4. Experimental results

We employ sample ECG data from several databases to perform our experimental study: the CinC Challenging Data as referenced in Ref. [2] (also known as the Physionet challenge dataset in Ref. [21]), a noninvasive fetal ECG database in Ref. [19], sample ECG sequences from MIT-BIS Arrhythmia Dataset [8], and some synthetic ECG data from Dr. Igal A. Sebag's example [39]. The main set of experiments with demographic data on sample patients with clinical/synthetic information were summarized in **Table 1**.

The first set of experiments mainly recorded the quantitative evaluations on several representative noninvasive FECG detection schemes based on single-channel abdominal ECG recordings. We studied the test by Panigrahy and Sahu [19] where the QRS complex of FECG displays the most visible features after the preprocessing step of eliminating baseline wander and power line interference from MECG, then each scheme using noninvasive FECG database was implemented to test the detection performance within 60 s of measuring *R* waves.

The numerical results for SE, PPV, *F*-score, and DER on nine methods for FECG detection are illustrated in **Table 2**, where the first column chronologically enumerated the tested FECG detection schemes which correspond to the average score on each measure for the recorded R waves, and the last column specified the range of accuracy over a certain length of time duration [2, 19, 21].

From **Table 2**, we justify that the SE metric on eight FECG detection schemes achieved over 90% except the TA scheme; the metrics of PPV and *F*-score on seven schemes reached over 90% except for SVD and TA; regarding DER, SVD shows the worst performance while it is still as low as 18.7%. Among all the five parameters on the referred quantitative analysis, EKS + ANFIS displays the best overall scores for each metric, while EKF + ANFIS indicates the second best results on *F*-score, DER, and other range of accuracy.

http://dx.doi.org/10.5772/intechopen.69920

Datasets	Techniques	Demographic data	Comments
Set 1: CinC Challenging [2]; and Set 2: Noninvasive FECG databases [19]	Nine schemes on noninvasive FECG detection	Set 1: 10 pregnant women, ages ranging from 21 to 33 years (27.1 ± 4.3 years), gestational age: 20–28 weeks (25.0 ± 2.5 weeks). Set 2: Uncertain number of patients, gestational age: 21–40 weeks	Set 1: Comprises of 24 clinically acquired abdominal recordings (20-min each), healthy and pathological patients were both present while no ectopic beats detected for either mother or fetus. Set 2: Includes 55 multichannel ECG recordings
Set 3: MIT-BIS Arrhythmia database	Both linear and twin-*R* correlative predictors; (4, 2) LWT compression; GM(1, 1) grey prediction	Set 3: Sequential ECG data on 25 men aged 32–89 years and 22 women aged 23–89 years were included in the subjects, in which approximately 60% were inpatients.	Set 3: Contains a sum of 48 half-hour excerpts of two-channel, 24-hour ECG recordings selected from 47 subjects (there are two records from the same subject) studied by the BIH Arrhythmia Laboratory at MIT in 1975–1979.
Set 4 and Set 5: both samples on synthetic maternal and fetal ECG data;	Adaptive least-mean-square (LMS) or recursive-least-square (RLS) noise cancellation; dynamic thresholding	Set 4: Provides no specific details on the average gestational age, typically in the third trimester (28–40 weeks), normal pregnancy; Set 5: Gestational age of fetus are ~40 weeks (right before delivery), including samples of physiological and pathological fetus.	Set 4: Synthetic data simulating maternal heart rate of 80–90 bpm with peak voltage 3.5 millivolts and fetal heart rate distributed from 120 to 160 bpm with peak voltage ~0.2 millivolts. Set 5: similar synthetic data with maternal heart rate of 65–85 bpm and fetal heart rate of 110–150 bpm and T/QRS range of 0.05–0.1 [43].

Table 1. Summary on the main set of experiments for noninvasive techniques on ECG detection and monitoring.

Detection scheme	SE (%)	PPV (%)	*F*-score (%)	DER (%)	Range of accuracy (%)
SVD	90.2	89.2	89.7	18.7	70.6–88.3
EKF	91.5	93.3	92.4	14.2	78.1–97.5
TS	92.0	90.9	91.5	15.7	71.3–91.9
Nonparametric	93.2	92.1	92.7	13.7	79.1–92.3
EKS	92.6	93.6	93.1	13.0	79.1–92.5
TA	86.3	85.5	85.9	16.9	74.8–93.1
EKF + ANFIS	92.8	94.9	93.8	11.8	81.1–94.2
EKS + ANFIS	93.8	96.0	94.9	9.80	83.8–97.6
CS-based ICA	92.5	92.0	92.2	16.5	80.2–96.4

Table 2. Quantitative scores of average SE, PPV, F-score, DER, and range of accuracy on noninvasive FECG detection schemes using a sample FECG database (duration = 60 s).

The second set of experiments was conducted by using the standard database on MIT-BIS Arrhythmia [8] with some original sample data of mixed MECG and FECG. We first investigate the predicted output of errors in comparison to real data from a mixed ECG sequence. **Figure 4** displays four subplots, where (a) depicts an original sequence in time interval [0:1600]

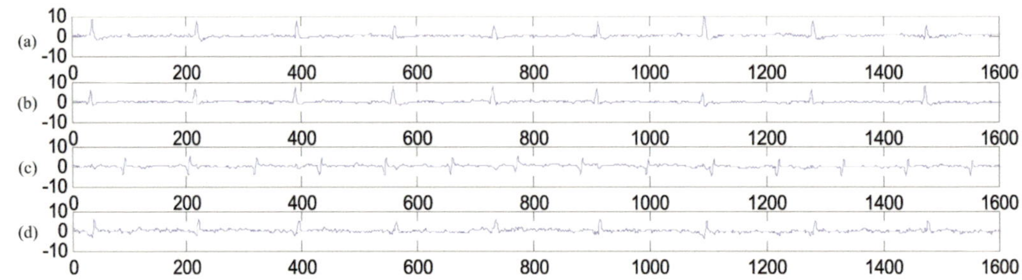

Figure 4. (a) Originally detected FECG; sequential data output by: (b) single linear prediction; (c) fourth-order linear prediction; (d) twin-*R* correlative prediction. Peak voltage denotes the location of *R* waves.

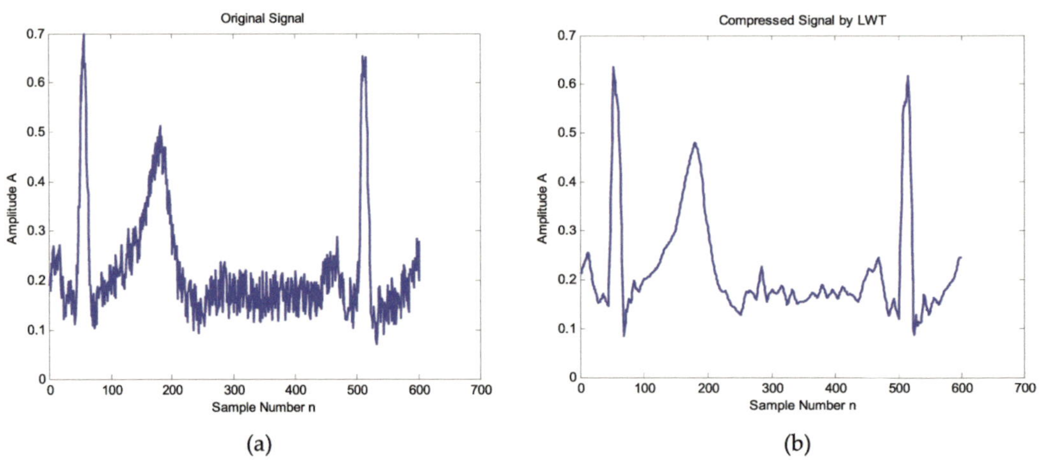

Figure 5. Proposed scheme: (a) original samples (SNR = 10 dB); (b) compressed output via (4, 2) LWT.

of the extracted FECG, (b) illustrates the first-order linear prediction, (c) presents the fourth-order linear prediction, and (d) shows the output of twin-*R* correlative prediction. We justify that the fourth-order predictor contains more false detections but less average errors comparing to the first-order predictor, while the proposed twin-*R* correlation predictor shows reduced average errors in contrast to the former two linear predictors [8].

We applied LWT for sequential ECG compression in time interval [400:1000] with additive random white noise (fmSNR = −10 dB). **Figure 5** displays the original ECG and its compressed output. Comparing **Figure 5(b)** to **Figure 5(a)**, we justify that the compressed ECG preserved most details of the original data with mild penalty of energy lost in the amplitude which comes from the quantization error as well as the loss from round-off decomposition in LWT.

Let us employ the compression ratio (CR) and percent root mean-square difference (PRD) [8, 12] to measure the quantitative compression performance on sequential ECE data: the tests as described below randomly selected 24 cases out of 48 from MIT-BIS Arrhythmia Database as testing samples. The proposed scheme recorded PRDs in a range of variable CRs with different quantization coefficients in comparison to those obtained by the Sabah's method.

	CR	2.0	3.0	5.0	7.0	9.0
PRD	Sabah	2.10	3.22	4.71	6.09	7.68
	Proposed	1.49	1.81	2.75	3.78	5.01
	CR	11.0	13.0	15.0	17.0	19.0
PRD	Sabah	9.33	11.1	12.3	14.0	16.8
	Proposed	6.32	7.67	9.20	11.3	13.6

Table 3. PRD comparison: the proposed scheme versus Sabah's.

We averaged each numerical value of PRD that corresponds to different CR, and enumerated the numbers on both the two schemes in **Table 3**. From the column comparison, we justify that by gaining the same CR ranging from 2.0 to 19.0, our scheme achieved much smaller PRDs than those of Sabah's, which suggests availability of achieving lower distortion rate by the proposed correlative prediction.

While the CR is under determination for both schemes on compression, let us consider CR as time points and PRD as the sequential output, a GM(1, 1) for the "time-sequence" T_1, T_2 is now constructed in order to obtain the predictive value of PRDs. From Eqs. (14) to (16), we are able to justify the positive correlativity between T_1 and T_2. From Eqs. (17) to (20), the solution to predictive GM(1, 1) model after LS updates and iterations is formulated as [8]:

$$T_1: \quad {T_1}^{(1)}(k+1) = (2.10 - 328.91)e^{-0.0026784k} + 328.91 \tag{28}$$

$$T_2: \quad {T_2}^{(1)}(k+1) = (1.49 - 150.95)e^{-0.0049531k} + 150.95 \tag{29}$$

Table 4 illustrates each value of the predicted PRDs obtained by our scheme versus Sabah's in condition of "extrapolated" and "interpolated" CRs. From column comparison, we justify that the GM(1, 1) prediction model performs well for the "extrapolated" CRs and presents closer predicted results in contrast with those of real PRD values in **Table 3**; most notably, if CRs become large enough, higher order polynomial fittings can be less reliable than predicting the "interpolated" time points while the functional fittings make less sense for extrapolated points, that is an auxiliary reason for using the gray system model on prediction.

	CR	4.0	8.0	12.0	16.0	20.0
PRD	Sabah	3.85	7.31	10.7	14.1	17.5
	Proposed	2.96	5.87	8.24	11.5	14.2
	CR	21.0	23.0	25.0	27.0	29.0
PRD	Sabah	18.3	20.0	21.6	23.3	24.9
	Proposed	14.9	16.3	17.6	18.9	20.2

Table 4. Predicted PRD (by GM(1,1)) of the proposed scheme versus Sabah's.

The third set of experiments illustrates the simulations of extracting FECG from MECG with additive noise with an adaptive least mean square (LMS) noise canceller to perform this task, which are depicted in **Figure 6** as modified from Dr. Igal A. Sebag's example [39] on both maternal and fetal heartbeat detections using sample synthetic ECG data. The six subplots permuted in the top row and in the middle row of **Figure 6** show the measuring procedure till the recovery of fetal heartbeat, where the convergence of adaptive noise cancellation takes up to 5–6 s on average. With the assumptions on a sampling rate of 4000 Hz and time duration of 40 s, the maternal heart rate is 89 beats per minute (bpm), and the fmSNR is adjusted as approximately −11.5 dB so as to simulate a test example on the third trimester of pregnancy. The fetal heart rate (FHR) is apparently faster than that of the mother's, normally ranging from 120 to 160 bpm and descending with the progress of gestational weeks. Since the measured FECG via abdominal recordings is often dominated by the maternal heartbeat signal propagating from the chest cavity to maternal abdomen, such path of propagation is constructed as a finite impulse response (FIR) filter with 10 randomized coefficients, with uncorrelated additive random noise which is 0.02 time of the original signal. While the reference signal of MECG is still surrounded with noise, an adaptive LMS filter with 15 coefficients and a step size of 0.00007 can be applied for simplicity of use. Note that the remainder of the error signal after the convergence of the system indicates an estimate of the fetal heartbeat signal associated with the measurement noise.

The bottom row of **Figure 6** comprises three subplots, where the left one shows the filtered FECG in contrast to its reference, the middle one indicates peak detection by applying dynamic thresholds to the filtered FECG and using vertical lines to mark each peak on any FECG signal

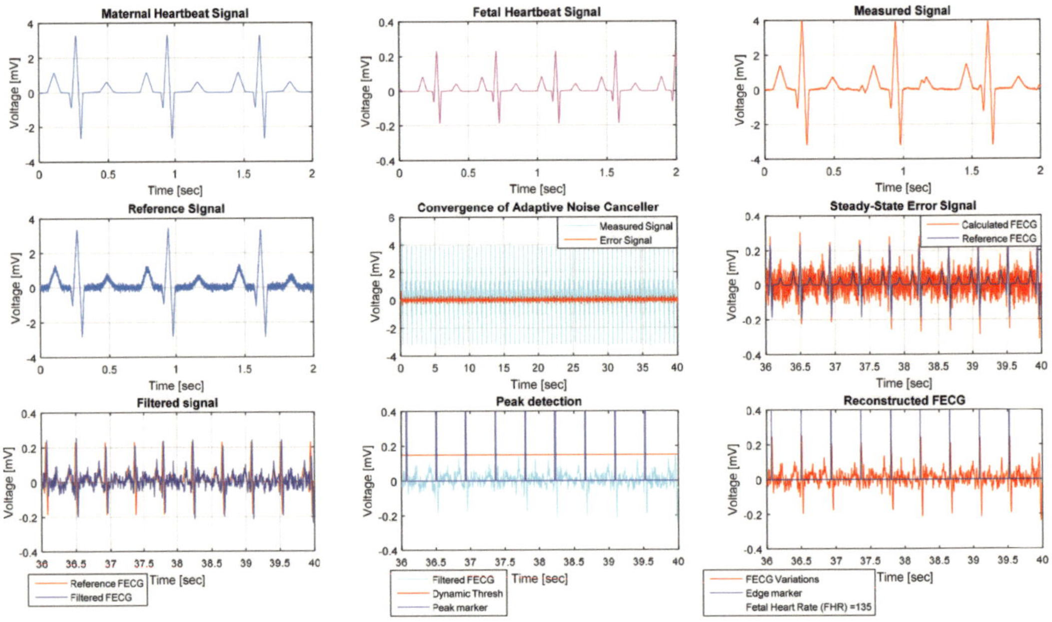

Figure 6. Automatic fetal heart rate detection on the reconstructed FECG from the original heartbeat signals of both mother and fetus.

crossing the threshold, and the right one depicts the reconstructed FECG data with variations and the automatically calculated FHR equals 135 bpm during the time interval of 36–40 s, which coincides with those normal diagnostic examples in FHR monitoring before delivery.

The experiments were conducted and retested via the software platform of MATLAB R2011a and higher versions in a Dell laptop with Core i7-4500U 1.80G CPU and 8GB RAM. We plan to include some specific analysis on the single-channel recordings for both healthy and pathological patients during the second and third trimester of pregnancy, and how the theoretical noninvasive FECG extraction algorithms influence the reconstruction accuracy of ECG signals from clinical experiments in later investigations.

Simulations on a real-life monitoring case were included in the two diagrams of **Figure 7**, where the occurrence of a typical scene on fetal hypoxia was illustrated in types of two parameters such as FHR (ranging from 70 to 150 bpm) and T/QRS (30 samples) in a 10-min

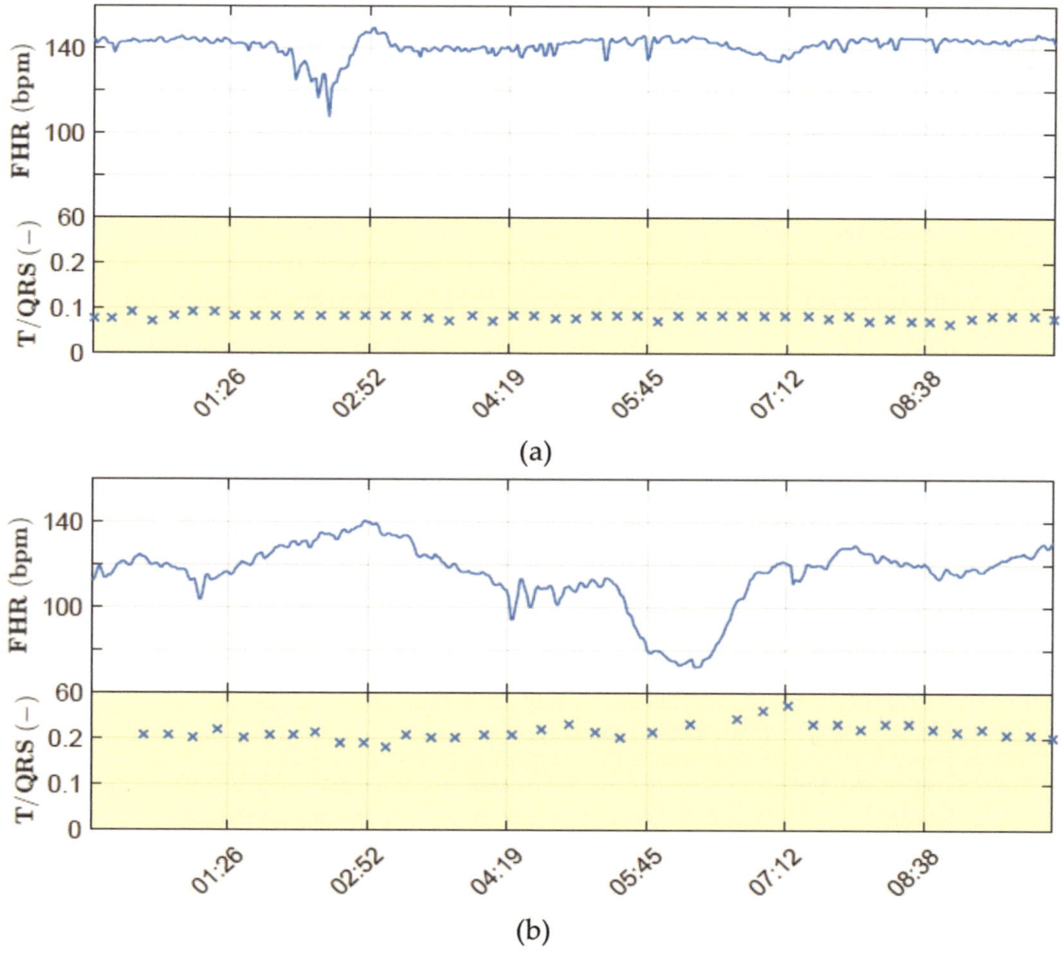

Figure 7. Simulations of sample data on FHR and T/QRS [43] in a 10-min time sequence for cases of: (a) physiological recordings (top); and (b) pathological recordings (bottom).

recording [43]. The top diagram and the bottom diagram depict recordings of a physiological sample and a pathological sample, respectively. Relatively steady FHR in **Figure 7(a)** indicates fetus in good condition, while the large valley in the waveform of FHR (especially at around the time of minute 06:00) in **Figure 7(b)** exhibits the abnormal oscillations of fetal heartbeats resulting from intrauterine hypoxia. For the physiological sample, the parameters are comparatively stable in which FHR displays fluctuations around 140 bpm at most of the time and T/QRS indicates minor numerical vibrations around 0.1; for the pathological sample, FHR exhibits larger amplitude of oscillations ranging from 70 to 140 bpm, while the numerical value of balance point on T/QRS fluctuations is around 0.2. In this trial, it is concluded that the value of fmSNR represents the most crucial factor affecting the quality of filtration, while both the parameter settings on the adaptive filtering system and the locations of electrodes contribute to the signal outputs on abdominal recordings [43].

5. Conclusions

A concise study of recent noninvasive FECG detection schemes has been established in this chapter. We have investigated a variety of algorithms for both single-channel and multichannel noninvasive FECG separation from MECG in abdominal recordings. The extended Kalman-based approach with algorithm variations modeled nonlinearity in single-channel cases, achieved considerably good performance on both synthetic and real-life ECG data. The extended Kalman smoother with ANFIS displays the best overall results on the set of performance metrics among nine noninvasive methods for FECG detection.

We have proposed a scheme of twin-*R* correlative prediction by applying (4, 2) LWT that effectively exploits correlation characteristics of time-domain ECG for sequential data processing. We have feasibly realized the parameter evaluation of ECG compression by building up a predictive GM(1, 1) model in order to give solutions to PRDs with both extrapolated and interpolated CRs, and achieved lower distortion rates in contrast to those of Sabah's. The correlation predictor with the multivariable gray model displays validity and efficiency for compression, suggesting a prospective technique for ECG data prediction and parameter evaluation. The modified simulation trials on fetal heartbeat detection by reconstructing FECG from maternal abdominal recordings via adaptive noise cancellation, provide an example on automatic FHR estimation on synthetic ECG data [39]; sample trials for either physiological case or pathological case on FHR recordings with modeling of hypoxia on mature fetus were included and reported in adaptive control systems for noninvasive monitoring [43].

As future work, we plan to improve one of the recent noninvasive FECG detection schemes by collaborating high-order dimensional data mining (i.e., inducing robust tensor decompositions to the dynamic filter-based models) to the ICA-based JADE scheme for FECG extraction from multichannel abdominal recordings, and updating the prediction system via statistical machine learning other than ANFIS, where the cocktail party-based solutions suggest a feasible tool for technical improvements [40]. We also plan to design an analytical software platform using the wavelet toolbox, which is oriented for detecting fetal cardiac arrhythmias with more practical trials on real data toward the multilead system for abdominal ECG recordings.

Author details

Xin Gao

Address all correspondence to: xgao1985@email.arizona.edu

Department of Electrical and Computer Engineering, the University of Arizona, Tucson, USA

References

[1] Adithya PC, Sankar R, Moreno WA, Hart S. Trends in fetal monitoring through phonocardiography: Challenges and future directions. Biomedical Signal Processing and Control. 2017;**33**:289–305

[2] Andreotti F, Riedl M, Himmelsbach T, Wedekind D, Wessel N, Stepan H, Schmieder C, Jank A, Malberg H, Zaunseder S. Robust fetal ECG extraction and detection from abdominal leads. Physiological Measurement. 2014;**35**(8):1551–1568

[3] Assaleh K. Extraction of fetal electrocardiogram using adaptive neuro-fuzzy interference systems. IEEE Transactions on Biomedical Engineering. 2007;**54**(1):59–68

[4] Behar J, Johnson A, Clifford GD, Oster J. A comparison of single channel fetal ECG extraction methods. Annals of Biomedical Engineering. 2014;**42**(6):1340–1353

[5] Behar J, Oster J, Clifford GD. Non-invasive FECG extraction from a set of abdominal sensors. In: IEEE Conference of Computing in Cardiology (CinC); September 22–24; Zaragoza, Spain. IEEE; 2013. pp. 197–200

[6] Clifford GD, Sameni R, Ward J, Robinson J, Wolfberg AJ. Clinically accurate fetal ECG parameters acquired from maternal abdominal sensors. American Journal of Obstetrics and Gynecology. 2011;**205**(1):47.e1–47.e5

[7] Clifford GD, Silva I, Behar J, Moody GB. Non-invasive fetal ECG analysis. Physiological Measurement. 2014;**35**(8):1521–1536

[8] Gao X. On the improved correlative prediction scheme for aliased electrocardiogram (ECG) data compression. In: 2012 Annual International Conference of the IEEE Engineering in Medicine and Biology Society (EMBC); August 28-September 01; San Diego, CA, USA. 2012. pp. 6180–6183

[9] Ghodsi M, Hassani H, Sanei S. Extracting fetal heart signal from noisy maternal ECG by singular spectrum analysis. Journal of Statistics and its Interface, Special Issue on the Application of SSA. 2010;**3**(3):399–411

[10] Hyvarinen A. Fast and robust fixed-point algorithms for independent component analysis. IEEE Transactions on Neural Networks. 1999;**10**(3):626–634

[11] Immanuel JJR, Prabhu V, Christopheraj VJ, Sugumar D, Vanathi PT. Separation of maternal and fetal ECG signals from the mixed source signal using FASTICA. Procedia Engineering. 2012;**30**:356–363

[12] Jafari MG, Chambers JA. Fetal electrocardiogram extraction by sequential source separation in the wavelet domain. IEEE Transactions on Biomedical Engineering. 2005;**52** (3):390–400

[13] Jalaleddine SMS, Hutehens CG, Strattan RD, Coberly WA. ECG data compression techniques−−A unified approach. IEEE Transactions on Biomedical Engineering. 1990;**37** (4):329–343

[14] Kropfl M, Modre-Osprian R, Schreier G, Hayn D. A robust algorithm for fetal QRS detection using non-invasive maternal abdominal ECGs. Computing in Cardiology. 2013;**40**:313–316

[15] Kumar P, Sharma SK, Prasad S. Detection of FECG from multivariate abdominal recordings using wavelets and neuro-fuzzy systems. International Journal of Engineering and Advanced Technology Studies. 2013;**2**(1):45–51

[16] Lathauwer L, Moor B, Vanderwalle J. Fetal electrocardiogram extraction by blind source subspace separation. IEEE Transactions on Biomedical Engineering. 2000;**47**(5):567–572

[17] Guerrero-Martinez JF, Martinez-Sober M, Bataller-Mompean M, Magdalena-Benedito JR. New algorithm for fetal QRS detection in surface abdominal records. Computers in Cardiology. 2006;**33**:441–444

[18] Melillo P, Santoro D, Vadursi M. Detection and compensation of inter-channel time offsets in indirect fetal ECG sensing. IEEE Sensors Journal. 2014;**14**(7):2327–2334

[19] Panigrahy D, Sahu PK. Extraction of fetal electrocardiogram (ECG) by extended state Kalman filtering and adaptive neuro-fuzzy inference system (ANFIS) based on single channel abdominal recording. Sadhana. 2015;**40**(Part 4):1091–1104

[20] Peters CHL, Van Laar JOEH, Vullings R, Oei SG, Wijn PFF. Beat-to-beat heart rate detection in multi-lead abdominal fetal ECG recordings. Medical Engineering & Physics. 2012;**34**(3):333–338

[21] Poian GD, Bernardini R, Rinaldo R. Separation and analysis of fetal-ECG signals from compressed sensed abdominal ECG recordings. IEEE Transactions on Biomedical Engineering. 2016;**63**(6):1269–1279

[22] Reza S, Shamsollahi MB, Jutten C, Clifford GD. A nonlinear Bayesian filtering framework for ECG denoising. IEEE Transactions on Biomedical Engineering. 2007;**54**(12):2172–2185

[23] Rooijakkers MJ, Rabotti C, de Lau H, Oei SG, Bergmans JWM, Mischi M. Feasibility study of a new method for low-complexity fetal movement detection from abdominal ECG recordings. IEEE Journal of Biomedical and Health Informatics. 2016;**20**(5):1361–1368

[24] Rosén KG, Amer-Wåhlin I, Luzietti R, Norén H. Fetal ECG waveform analysis. Best Practice & Research Clinical Obstetrics & Gynaecology. 2004;**18**(3):485–514

[25] Rosén KG, Samuelsson A. Device for reducing signal noise in a fetal ECG signal. U.S. Patent 6658284, issued December 2, 2003

[26] Santiago MC. Processing of Abdominal Recordings by Kalman Filters [Internet]. 2012. Available from: https://upcommons.upc.edu/bitstream/handle/2099.1/16148/Final_Project_Marcos_Cruz_Processing_of_abdominal_recordings_by_Kalman_filters.pdf

[27] Selvaraj R, Kanagaraj B. A multi-stage adaptive singular value decomposition approach for fetal ECG signal extraction in multichannel input system for prenatal health monitoring. Asian Journal of Information Technology. 2016;**15**(6):1049–1055

[28] Silva I, Behar J, Sameni R, Zhu T-T, Oster J, Clifford GD, Moody GB. Noninvasive fetal ECG: The PhysioNet/computing in cardiology challenge 2013. In: IEEE Conference of Computing in Cardiology (CinC); September 22–24. 2013. pp. 149–152

[29] Song S, Rooijakkers MJ, Harpe P, Rabotti C, Mischi M, van Roermund AHM, Cantatore E. A noise reconfigurable current-reuse resistive feedback amplifier with signal-dependent power consumption for fetal ECG monitoring. IEEE Sensors Journal. 2016;**16**(23):8304–8313

[30] Tadi MJ, Lehtonen E, Hurnanen T, Koskinen J, Eriksson J, Pänkäälä M, Teräs M, Koivisto T. A real-time approach for heart rate monitoring using a Hilbert transform in seismocardiograms. Physiological Measurement. 2016;**37**(11):1885–1909

[31] Taylor MJO, Smith MJ, Thomas M, Green AR, Cheng F, Oseku-Afful S, Wee L-Y, Fisk NM, Gardiner HM. Non-invasive fetal electrocardiography in singleton and multiple pregnancies. BJOG: An International Journal of Obstetrics & Gynaecology. 2003;**110**(7):668–678

[32] Yeh H-M, Chang Y-C, Lin C, Yeh C-H, Lee C-N, Shyu M-K, Hung M-H, et al. A new method to derive fetal heart rate from maternal abdominal electrocardiogram monitoring fetal heart rate during cesarean section. PLoS One. 2015;**10**(2):e0117509

[33] Yu S-H. Detection of fetal cardiac repolarization abnormalities using magneto-cardiography [Ph.D. Dissertation]. The University of Wisconsin-Madison; 2013

[34] Zarzoso V, Nandi AK. Noninvasive fetal electrocardiogram extraction blind separation versus adaptive noise cancellation. IEEE Transactions on Biomedical Engineering. 2001;**48** (1):12–20

[35] Zheng W, Li X-L, Wei X-Y, Liu H-X. Foetal ECG extraction by support vector regression. Electronic Letters. 2016;**52**(7):506–507

[36] Zheng W, Wei X-Y, Zhong J-J, Liu H-X. Fetal heart beat detection by Hilbert transform and non-linear state-space projections. IET Science, Measurement & Technology. 2015;**9** (1):85–92

[37] Zhong Y-D. Blind adaptive filtering for extraction of fetal ECG from maternal abdominal ECG [Ph.D. Dissertation]. The University of Illinois at Chicago; 2007

[38] https://en.wikipedia.org/wiki/Data_compression_ratio

[39] https://www.mathworks.com/matlabcentral/fileexchange/35328-simulink-model-for-fetal-ecg-extraction--hdl-compatible-algorithm-/content/mom_and_fetus.m

[40] https://cran.r-project.org/web/packages/JADE/vignettes/JADE-BSSasymp.pdf

[41] https://www.cablesandsensors.com/pages/12-lead-ecg-placement-guide-with-llustrations

[42] Lynn WD, Escalona OJ, McEneaney DJ. Arm and wrist surface potential mapping for wearable ECG rhythm recording devices: A pilot clinical study. Sensors & their Applications, Journal of Physics: Conference Series. 2013;**450**:012026. DOI: 10.1088/1742-6596/450/1/012026; http://iopscience.iop.org/article/10.1088/1742-6596/450/1/012026/pdf

[43] Martinek R, Kahankova R, Nazeran H, Konecny J, Jezewski J, Janku P, Bilik P, Zidek J, Nedoma J, Fajkus M. Non-invasive fetal monitoring: A maternal surface ECG electrode placement-based novel approach for optimization of adaptive filter control parameters using the LMS and RLS algorithms. Sensors. 2017;**17**(5):1154. http://www.mdpi.com/1424-8220/17/5/1154

Section 2

Understanding Electrograms from Cardiac Devices

Chapter 5

Pacemaker and ICD Troubleshooting

Sorin Lazar, Henry Huang and Erik Wissner

Additional information is available at the end of the chapter

http://dx.doi.org/10.5772/intechopen.69998

Abstract

Continuous advancements in technology and software algorithms for pacemakers and implantable cardioverter-defibrillators (ICDs) have improved functional reliability and broadened their diagnostic capabilities. At the same time, understanding management and troubleshooting of modern devices has become increasingly complex for the device implanter. This chapter provides an overview of the underlying physics and basic principles important to pacemaker and ICD function. The second part of this chapter outlines common device problems encountered in patients with pacemakers and ICDs and provides solutions and tips for troubleshooting.

Keywords: signal processing, filters, pacemaker troubleshooting, ICD troubleshooting

1. Introduction: Device physics

1.1. Signal processing

Signal processing refers to the science of analyzing time-varying physical processes [1]. Signal processing is divided into two categories: analog signal processing and digital signal processing. An analog signal is continuous in time and can take on a continuous range of amplitude values. A discrete-time signal is an independent time variable that is quantized so that only the value of the signal at the discrete instant in time is known. This can be illustrated in the following example: a continuous sinewave with peak amplitude of 1 and frequency of f is described in Eq. (1):

$$x(t) = \sin(2\pi f t) \tag{1}$$

where the frequency f is measured in Hertz (Hz).

By plotting Eq. (1) a continuous curve is obtained (**Figure 1a**). If the continuous waveform represents a continuous physical voltage sampling every t_s seconds, using an analog-to-digital converter would result in a sinewave represented as a sequence of discrete values shown in **Figure 1(b)**. **Figure 1(b)** represents the digitization of the continuous signal in **Figure 1(a)**. Variable t in Eq. (1) and **Figure 1(a)** is a continuous and independent variable. Variable n in **Figure 1(b)** is a discrete and independent variable that can take only integer values. As a result, the index n identifies the elements of the digital signal in **Figure 1(b)**. All naturally occurring intracardiac signals are continuous and all signals stored by pacemakers and defibrillators are digital.

1.2. Filtering

Filters are used for two general purposes: (1) separation of signals that have been combined and (2) restoration of signals that have been distorted in some form. Signal separation is needed when if the signal is contaminated by interference, noise or other signals. As an example, filtering is used to separate nonphysiologic high-frequency pulmonary vein potentials recorded during catheter ablation of atrial fibrillation (AF) from physiologic signals. Signal restoration is used

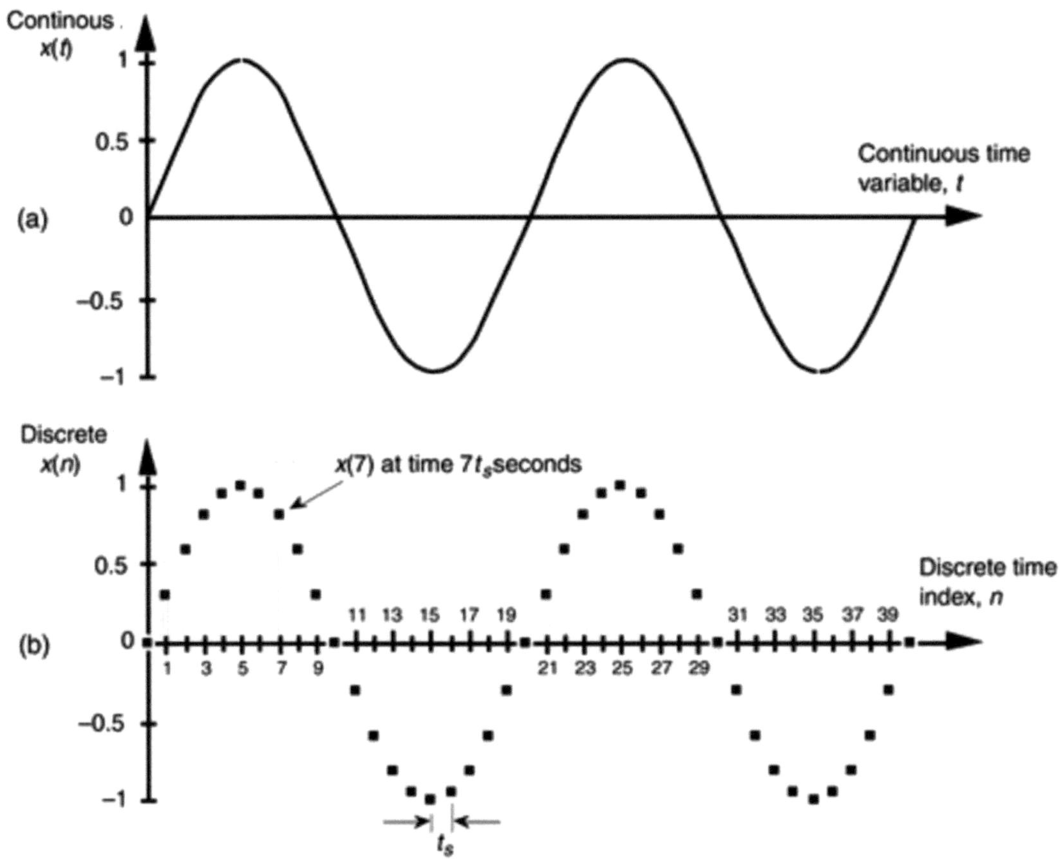

Figure 1. A time-domain sinewave: (a) continuous waveform representation and (b) discrete sample representation.

when a signal has been distorted in some form. For example, an audio recording obtained with poor equipment may be filtered to improve fidelity so the actual sound is better reproduced.

For raw signal data to be analyzed, information must be represented in either the time or frequency domain. The most commonly used filters applied in intracardiac devices are in the frequency domain. **Figure 2** summarizes the four most common basic frequency responses. These filters allow unaltered passing of some frequencies, while other frequencies are completely blocked. Those frequencies that pass through are called "passband," while frequencies that are blocked are referred to as "stopband." The band in-between is called the "transition band." A very narrow transition band is called "fast roll-off," "The cut-off frequency" is the frequency that separates the "passband" from the "transition band," Analog filters use a cut-off frequency that is decreased to 0.707 from the original amplitude. Digital filters are less strict, and usually the cut-offs used are 99, 90, 70.7, and 50% of the original amplitude levels.

The example shown in **Figure 3** highlights the three parameters described above. An example of a "fast roll-off," is shown in (a) and (b). A "passband ripple" example is shown in (c) and (d), and finally, "stopband attenuation" is shown in (e) and (f).

1.3. Chebyshev filters

Chebyshev filters are used to separate one band of frequencies from another. They are the most commonly used in cardiac electrophysiology applications. The primary attribute of Chebyshev filters is their speed. The Chebyshev response is a mathematical strategy for achieving a faster "roll-off" by allowing "ripple" in the frequency response.

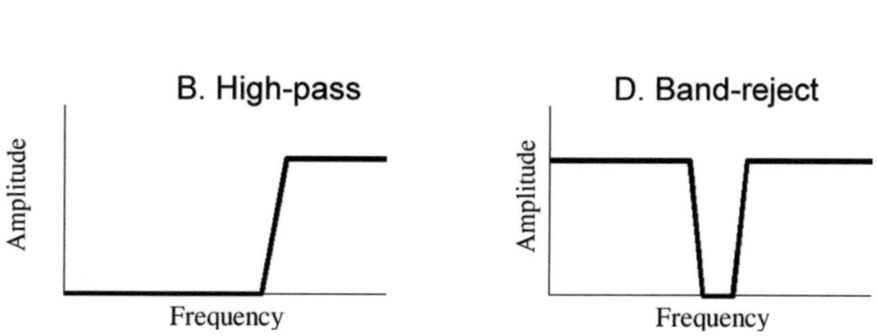

Figure 2. The four common frequency responses.

Figure 4 shows three ripple values, 0, 0.5, and 20%, for a low-pass Chebyshev filter. If the ripple decreases (good) the roll-off becomes less sharp (bad). The Chebyshev filter design is an optimal balance between these two parameters. If the ripple is 0%, the filter is called "Butterworth filter." A ripple of 0.5% is often a good choice for digital filters. This matches the typical precision and accuracy of the analog electronics that the signal has passed through.

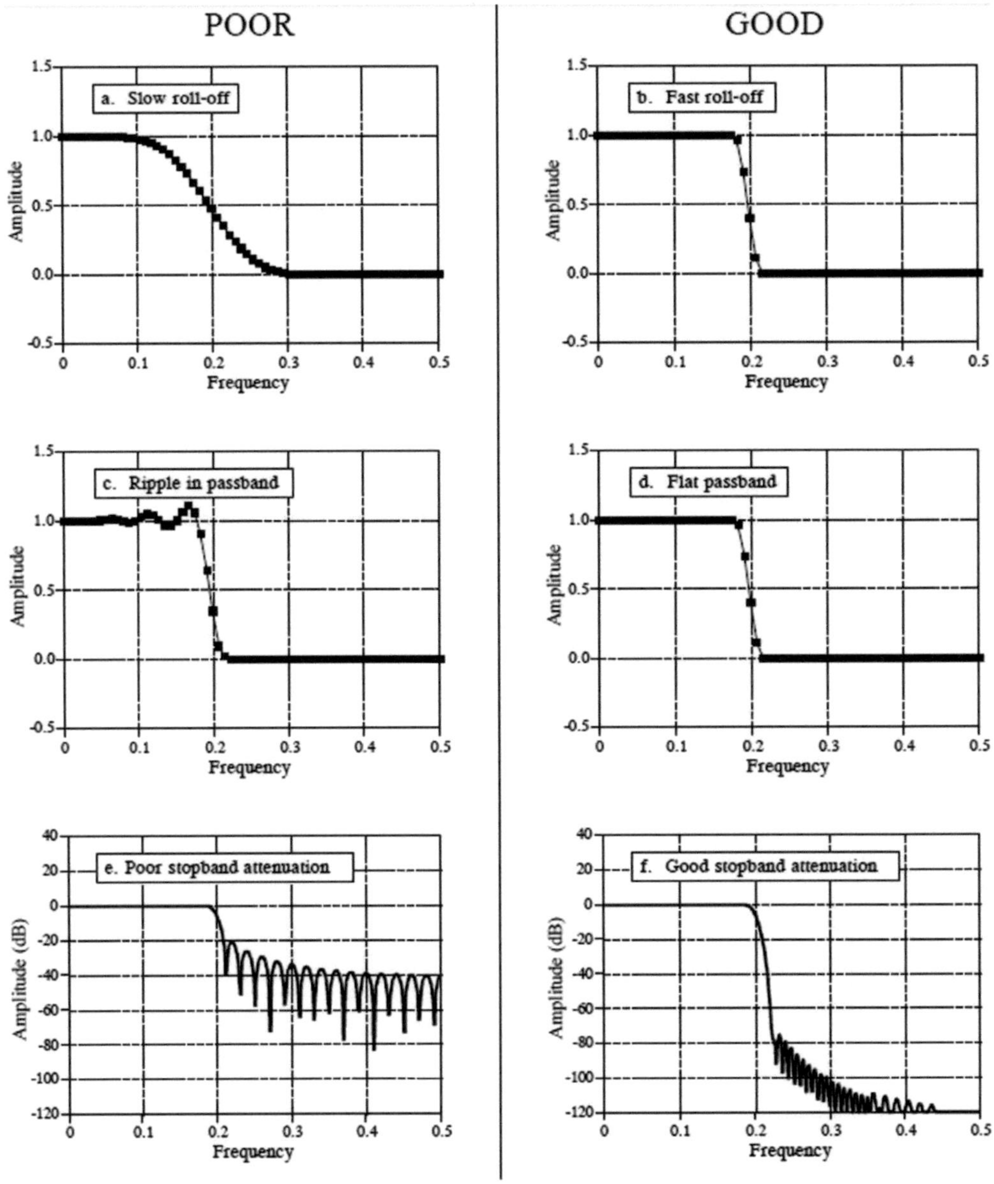

Figure 3. The three parameters important for evaluating frequency domain performance: (1) roll-off sharpness, (a) and (b); (2) passband ripple, (c) and (d); and (3) stopband attenuation, (e) and (f).

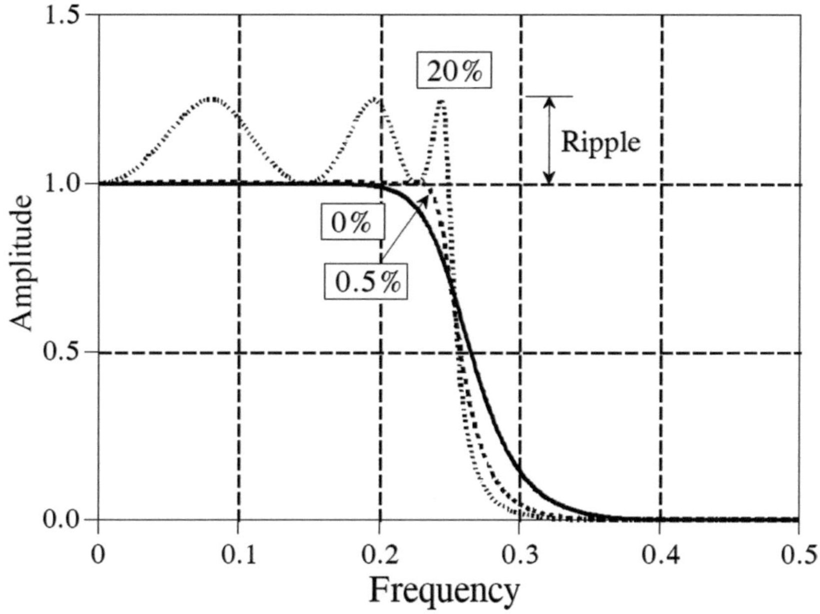

Figure 4. The Chebyshev response: Chebyshev filters achieve a faster roll-off by allowing ripple in the passband. When the ripple is set to 0%, it is called a maximally flat or Butterworth filter.

1.4. Unipolar versus bipolar recordings

All electrical circuits must have a cathode (negative pole) and an anode (positive pole) [2]. In general, there are two types of electrical circuits used in pacing systems depending on the location of the anode. In a unipolar system, as shown in **Figure 5(a)**, the metal can of the pacemaker is used as the anode (+), and the distal electrode of pacemaker lead as the cathode (−). In a unipolar system, the pacing lead has only one electrical pole. **Figure 5(b)** shows the other type, a BIPOLAR system where both the anode (+) and cathode (−) are located on the same pacing lead. In all pacing systems, the distal pole that is in direct contact with cardiac tissue is negative. All currently available ICDs are bipolar, however, based on the lead utilized, the system may be dedicated bipolar or integrated bipolar. In a dedicated bipolar design, the anode is separate from the shock coil. In an integrated design, the distal shock coil also serves as the anode for pacing and sensing. An integrated design allows for more simple lead construction, as the distal shock coil serves two purposes. A dedicated bipolar system may provide more reliable sensing than an integrated design with a shared coil, as the anode is not affected by the high-voltage shock. Unipolar pacing systems have the advantage of a simpler and more reliable single-coil lead construction. It is also much easier to appreciate the pacing artifact of a unipolar system due to the anatomic distance between lead and pulse generator with parts of the electrical circuit closer to the skin surface. In some instances, sensing and capture thresholds are better than those obtained from a bipolar system, although lower lead impedance may result in higher current drain from the battery. In order to reduce the risk of pacemaker stimulation of the pectoralis muscle and/or device oversensing of electrical signals generated by the pectoralis muscle, many of the older pacemaker models incorporated a layer of protective coating on the device side facing the muscular tissue.

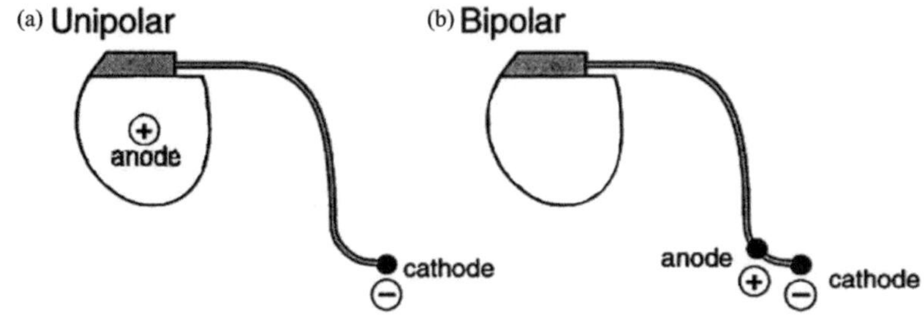

Figure 5. (a) Unipolar pacing system: the lead tip is the cathode and the pacemaker is the anode. (b) Bipolar pacing system: the lead tip is the cathode and the proximal ring is the anode. The pacemaker is not part of the circuit.

Bipolar pacing systems offer several advantages that have made this polarity choice increasingly popular, especially as dual-chamber pacing has become more prevalent in clinical practice. Because the distance between the individual electrodes is small (short antenna) and since both are located deep within the body, bipolar devices are less susceptible than unipolar systems to electrical interference caused by skeletal muscle activity or electromagnetic interference (EMI). Also, higher output settings required for unipolar pacing may result in stimulation of the pocket around the pacemaker. This problem is virtually unknown in normally functioning bipolar systems. One downside to using bipolar pacing is that the pacing artifact is very small and often difficult to discern on the surface electrocardiogram. This makes determination of proper function and malfunction more difficult. For this reason, it is not uncommon to see a pacemaker programmed to unipolar pacing but bipolar sensing.

1.5. Sensing

Sensing is the ability of the device to detect the intrinsic cardiac activity [3]. This is measured in millivolts (mV). The larger the signal in mV, the easier it is for the device to sense the event as well as to discriminate normal intrinsic from spurious electrical signals. Setting the sensitivity of a pacemaker is often confusing. When programming this value, it must be understood that the value programmed is the smallest amplitude signal that will be sensed (**Figure 6**). There is an inverse relation between sensing and sensitivity. The higher the sensing value, the lower the sensitivity to detect the intrinsic electrical signal. Thus, a setting of 8 mV requires at least an 8 mV electrical signal for the pacemaker to detect. A 2 mV setting will allow any signal above 2 mV to be sensed by the pacemaker.

1.6. Slew rate

Measurement of the intrinsic electrical signal for sensing is not simple, as the pacemaker does not use the entire electrical signal that is present. This "raw" electrical signal is filtered to eliminate a majority of noncardiac signals as well as portions of the cardiac signals that are not needed. Because filtering allows only certain frequencies to pass through to the sensing circuit, the final "filtered" signal may be substantially different from the original signal

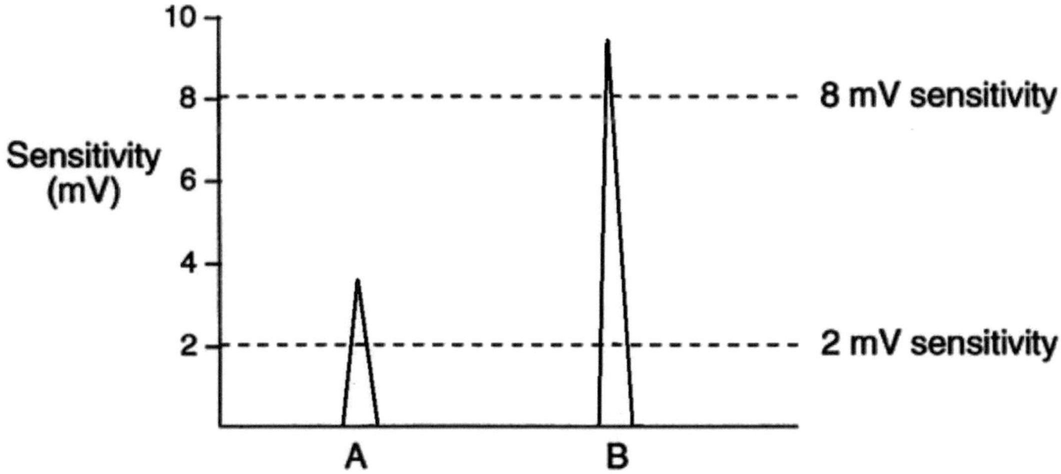

Figure 6. Concept of sensitivity. Electrogram A is 3 mV in size and electrogram B is 10 mV in size. At sensitivity of 2 mV, both electrical signals have sufficient amplitude to be sensed. At setting of 8 mV, only the larger signal will be sensed.

(**Figure 7**). One way of measuring the quality of a sensed signal is to look at the slew rate. The slew rate refers to the slope of the intrinsic signal (**Figure 8**) and is measured in volts/second. High slew rates (>1.0 V/s in the ventricle and >0.5 V/s in the atrium) are desirable for consistent sensing.

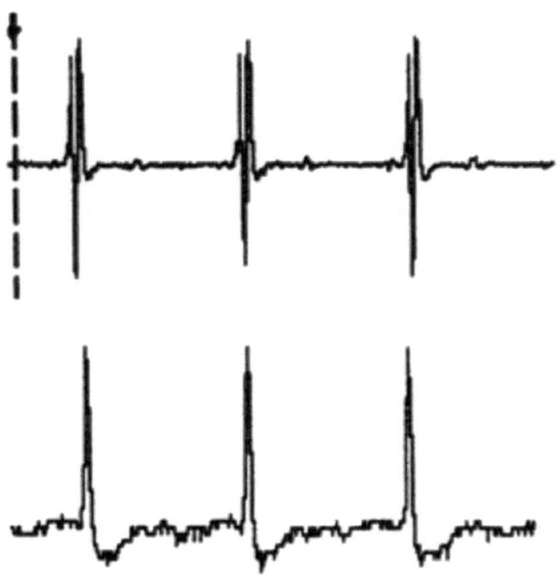

Figure 7. Raw and filtered electrograms sensed by a pacemaker. The top tracing is the filtered signal used by the pacemaker for sensing. Filtering of the raw signal is necessary to prevent (over)sensing of the T-wave, far-field signals, and myopotentials.

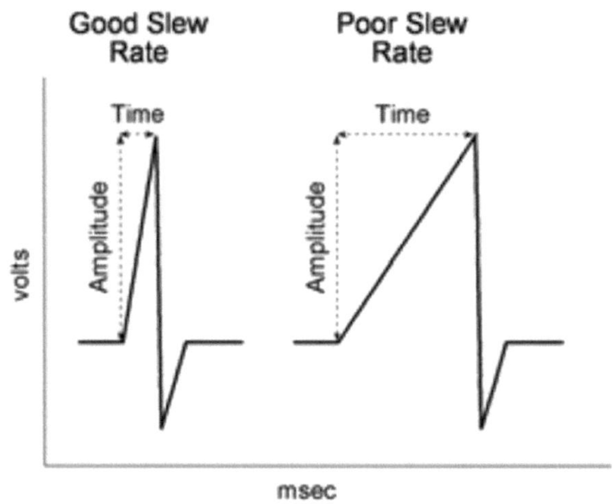

Figure 8. Slew rate measured in volt/second. The more rapid the voltage increase, the sharper the electrogram, the higher the slew rate.

1.7. Automaticity

As pacing systems become increasingly sophisticated, programming optimal pacing and sensing parameters for individual patients also becomes more difficult [4]. In addition, biological systems by nature are constantly changing, making settings that are appropriate at one point in time inappropriate at other times. Some pacemakers now have algorithms to automatically adjust one or more parameters. Automaticity is commonly applied to the rate response sensor function and sensitivity. There are different sensitivity adjusting algorithms for pacemakers and ICDs. For pacemakers, these algorithms assess the size of the sensed signal, and then attempt to provide a safety margin by adjusting the sensitivity. This tends to result in a less sensitive setting for the ventricle, as much of the time ventricular signals are very large. Lowering the susceptibility to EMI, it may in turn cause occasional undersensing of ectopic intrinsic beats. For a bipolar pacing system, the nominal ("out of the box") sensitivity settings are usually acceptable and rarely result in under- or oversensing. Some pacemakers utilize an automatic gain feature similar to that of ICDs, which differs from the automatic adjustment feature currently in use in that the programmed sensing values remain unaffected (**Figure 9**).

Sensing the intrinsic heart rate is very important as this is the primary method for the ICD to detect the presence of a tachycardia. Typically, true bipolar and integrated bipolar configurations are used, while unipolar pacing and sensing have no role in ICD programming. True bipolar sensing in ICDs uses the same methodology as for conventional pacing leads. The dedicated pacing and sensing cathode and anode are located toward the distal tip of the lead within the ventricle (**Figure 10a**) and kept separate from the high-voltage shocking circuit. In an integrated bipolar configuration, the lead tip serves as the cathode and the distal shocking coil as the anode (**Figure 10b**) allowing for simpler lead design. However, since the shock coil doubles as the sensing coil, suboptimal sensing may result immediately after a shock has been delivered. Normal sensing resumes shortly after shock delivery once physiologic cardiac depolarization has returned. Some devices use true bipolar sensing and integrated bipolar pacing to overcome this limitation. The use of standard sensing protocols applying fixed

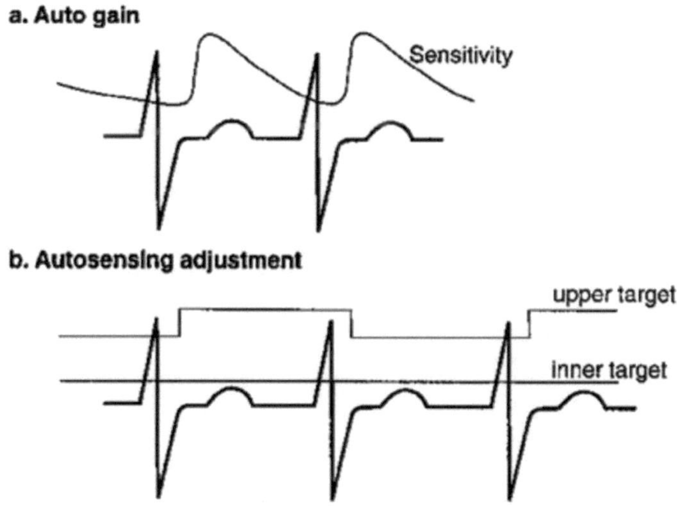

Figure 9. (a) Auto gain is a method to automate the sensing function. Sensitivity increases with the length of the sensing interval. Once a signal is sensed, the sensitivity abruptly decreases to avoid oversensing of the evoked response and the T-wave. (b) Autosensing adjustment is a method to automatically set the sensitivity. An inner and upper target is set for sensing. When a beat is sensed on both the inner and upper targets, the upper target is moved further out (made less sensitive) until sensing no longer occurs. The upper target is then moved back. In this way, the device can determine the signal amplitude and set the overall sensitivity of the device appropriately.

sensitivity values works well for pacemakers but not for ICDs because of the need to reliably sense and differentiate between varying clinically relevant rhythms such as sinus rhythm, premature ventricular (PVC) beats, and ventricular fibrillation where extreme variation in amplitude of intracardiac electrograms may occur. A fixed sensitivity level would be unable to adapt to these changes. Most ICDs use some variation of automatic sensitivity control, allowing for a "most sensitive value" to be programmed either as an absolute number or as a general term such as "least" or "most" sensitive. After a sensed event, the device reverts to higher sensing threshold in order to prevent T-wave oversensing or inadvertent oversensing of noncardiac

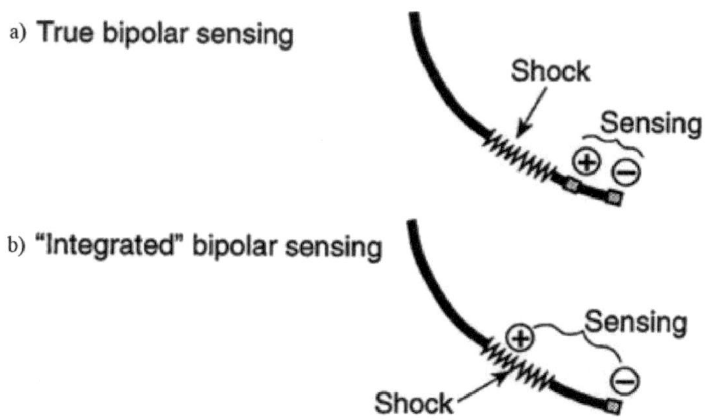

Figure 10. (a) True bipolar sensing occurs between the lead tip (cathode) and proximal ring (anode) independent of the defibrillation coil. (b) Integrated bipolar sensing utilizes the lead tip as the cathode and the defibrillation coil as the sensing anode. Sensing is more with a true bipolar configuration.

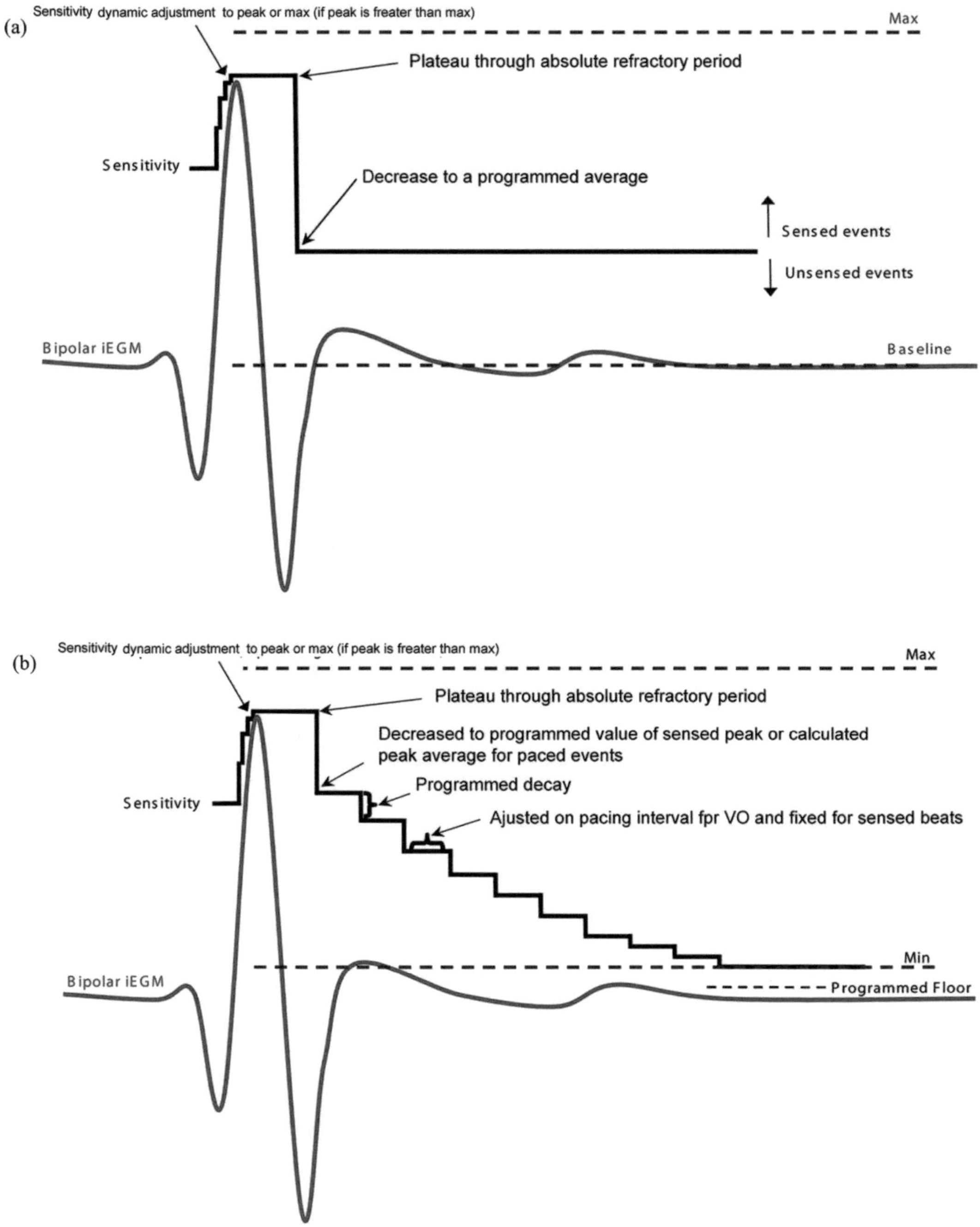

Figure 11. (a) A typical example of a bipolar right ventricular intracardiac electrogram from a pacemaker. The electrogram peak value is determined and the sensitivity is decreased to a fixed programmed value or a programmed average percentage of the peak value. (b) An example of a bipolar right ventricular intracardiac electrogram from a defibrillator. The electrogram peak value is determined and stored. Then a stepwise decay algorithm is used to the maximum programmed sensitivity. Sensitivity algorithms differ between device manufacturers.

http://dx.doi.org/10.5772/intechopen.69998

events. The longer the period the device monitors for a sensed event, the more sensitive it becomes. This function provides the ability to determine if the patient has gone into fine ventricular fibrillation that might otherwise be missed if the device was set at less sensitive settings. **Figure 11** shows a comparison of the sensing algorithms between pacemakers and ICDs.

2. Device troubleshooting

2.1. Pacemaker troubleshooting

The first step in evaluating pacemaker malfunction is to determine whether the function of the device is truly abnormal [5]. If a pacemaker malfunction has been confirmed, the next step consists of a detailed patient history. The history may provide important clues to the likely diagnosis. If the problem or complaint occurs shortly after device implant, lead dislodgment, loose set screws, misalignment of the lead within the connector block or poor lead placement should be suspected as potential causes [2]. In the acute period, battery depletion or lead fracture is highly unlikely. Conversely, a patient presenting with an older device is more likely to experience lead failure or battery depletion rather than lead dislodgment or connection issues.

A tachycardia driven by the pacemaker presents a more difficult situation. In most cases, application of a magnet or reprogramming the device will terminate the abnormal rhythm. In rare cases, the pacemaker will not respond to these simple measures, and urgent surgical intervention may be required for "runaway pacemaker" (**Figure 12**). This uncommon malfunction is caused by a major component failure in the pacing circuit. The vast majority of rapid ventricular-paced rhythms in Dual pacing, Dual sensing, Dual action (DDD) or Ventricular pacing, Dual sensing, Dual action (VDD) devices are due to tracking of atrial fibrillation or atrial flutter. The pacemaker will attempt to track the rapid atrial rate to the programmed upper rate limit (URL) if mode switching is not enabled or fails to respond appropriately. Placing a magnet over the device will drop the pacing rate to the magnet rate of the device until a nontracking mode such as DDI or Ventricular pacing, Ventricular sensing, Inhibited (VVI) is programmed. Sensor-driven devices may cause rapid pacing as well. After the patient is stabilized, a history is obtained, and the initial device data collected, the 12-lead surface Electrocardiogram (ECG) should be evaluated. An approach to determine the general function of the pacing system is detailed below:

i. Pacing

  a. Spike present

    1. Verify appropriate rate interval

    2. Verify appropriate depolarization response

      a. capture

      b. pseudo-fusion

      c. fusion

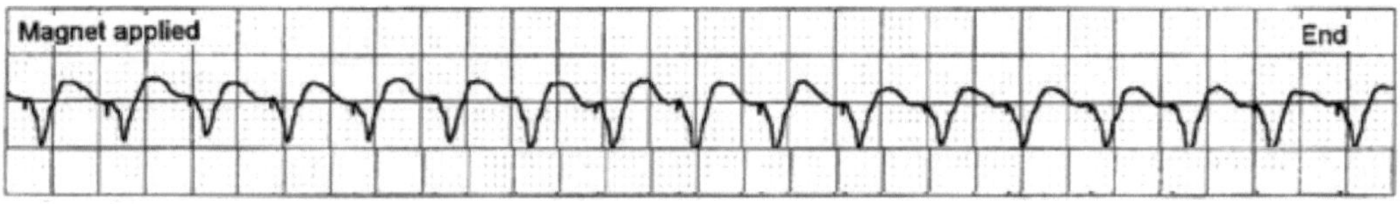

Figure 12. Runaway pacemaker: this strip shows VVI pacing at 180 bpm (the runaway protect limit on this device). The pacemaker was programmed to the DDD mode with an upper rate limit of 120 bpm. Therapeutic radiation delivered to the pacemaker in a patient with breast cancer resulted in circuit failure and rapid pacing. Even magnet application did not slow the pacing rate.

b. Spike absent

1. Apply magnet (magnet function must be enabled)

(Note: a ventricular pacemaker spike falling in the absolute refractory period of the myocardium will NOT result in capture.)

2. Observe for pace artifact and capture on 12-lead surface ECG.

ii. Sensing

a. Patient must have a nonpaced rhythm

b. Appropriate escape interval

iii. Compare function to known technical information, watch for end of service indicators and other variations

Oversensing is readily diagnosed by placing a magnet over the device. If the pacemaker was not pacing or paced too slow due to oversensing, pacing will resume once the magnet is in place. If there is no pacing with the magnet on, then either the pacemaker is not putting out a pulse or the pulse is not reaching the heart.

Causes for true pacemaker failure are noted below:

- Depletion of the device battery [6]
- Defibrillation close to or on top of the device
- Device in the radiation field [7]
- Devices on recall or alert with known modes of failure [8]
- Electrocautery use close to or on the device
- Random component failure
- Direct mechanical trauma to the device

2.1.1. Noncapture

This potentially life-threatening problem is identified by the presence of pacemaker pulse artifact without capture in the appropriate chamber following the impulse. Causes of noncapture are listed below [2]:

- Exit block (high capture threshold) or inappropriate programming resulting in insufficient output or pulse width
- Malfunction or inappropriate programming of automatic capture output algorithms
- Lead dislodgment
- Lead fracture
- Lead insulation failure
- Loose lead-to-pacemaker connection
- Low battery output
- Severe metabolic imbalance
- Threshold rise due to drug effect
- "Pseudo-noncapture" (pacing during the myocardial refractory period due to undersensing of the preceding complex)

2.1.1.1. *Corrective action*

Increase pacemaker output if possible. Where appropriate, revise or replace lead or pacemaker, correct metabolic imbalances. For pseudo-noncapture adjust the sensitivity to a more sensitive setting, or revise the lead if sensing is very poor. Program to unipolar polarity.

2.1.2. *Undersensing*

Undersensing is recognized by the presence of a pulse artifact that occurs after an intrinsic event, but fails to reset the escape interval. The pacing output may or may not capture depending on the timing during the cardiac cycle. Causes of undersensing (thus "overpacing") are listed below [9]:

- Poor lead position with poor R-wave or P-wave amplitude
- Lead dislodgment
- Lead fracture
- Lead insulation failure
- Lead perforation of the myocardium
- Severe metabolic disturbance
- Defibrillation near pacemaker
- Myocardial infarction of tissue near electrode
- Ectopic beats of low intracardiac amplitude

- Dual pacing, Ventricular sensing, Inhibited (DVI)-committed function
- Safety pacing
- Inappropriate programming
- Magnet application

2.1.2.1. Corrective action

Increase pacemaker sensitivity. Where appropriate, revise or replace the lead. Try reprogramming polarity. If the problem is very infrequent then careful observation may be acceptable.

2.1.3. Oversensing

A diagram highlighting the different components of a single-chamber pacemaker and ICD is shown in **Figure 13**. In a single-chamber system, oversensing is recognized by inappropriate inhibition of the pacemaker. Oversensing may result in total inhibition of output or prolongation of the escape interval. Myopotentials are a common cause of oversensing, which is seen predominately in unipolar pacemakers and usually results from sensing noncardiac muscle activity (e.g. pectoralis muscle or abdominal rectus muscles). Myopotentials are triggered by arm movements such as arm lifting in patients with prepectoral implants, or moving from a lying to sitting position in patients with abdominal implants. Oversensing may also occur if the ventricular lead falsely senses the T-wave. Despite an increase in environmental EMI, pacemakers prove fairly resistant to this type of interference because of continuous design improvements. Sensing intrinsic or extraneous EMI results in the device falsely detecting a cardiac event. The pacing output will be inhibited as long as these interfering signals continue. A dual-chamber system may track electrical signals such as myopotentials in either the atrium, ventricle or both. The atrial channel is usually set to a more sensitive value than the ventricular channel. Tracking may result from oversensing of electrical signals on the atrial channel, inhibiting atrial output, while these signals are too small to be sensed by the ventricular channel. Each time oversensing occurs on the atrial channel an atrioventricular interval (AVI) is triggered, resulting in ventricular output at a rate up to the programmed upper rate limit (URL). Causes of oversensing are listed below [9]:

- Myopotentials
- Electromagnetic interference
- T-wave sensing
- Far-field R-wave sensing (atrial lead)
- Lead insulation failure
- Lead dislodgement

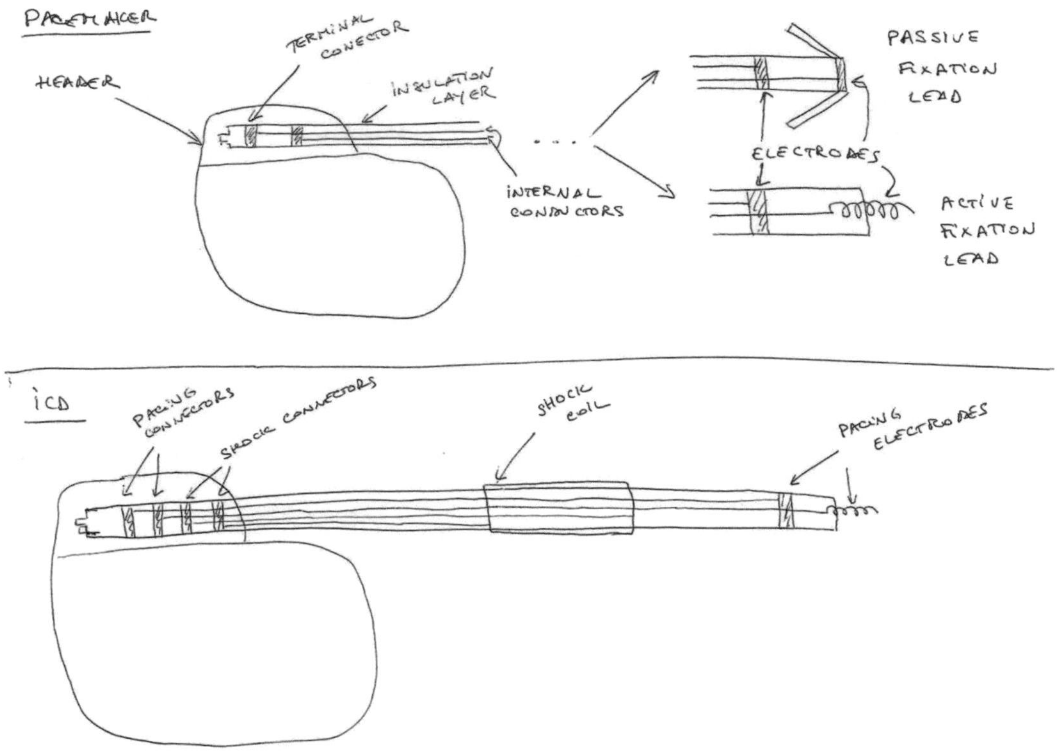

Figure 13. Basic components of a single-chamber pacemaker (top) and single-chamber ICD (bottom) (DF4 lead model shown).

- Lead fracture (**Image 1**)
- Loose fixation screw (**Image 2**)
- Crosstalk

2.1.3.1. Corrective action

Decrease the sensitivity of the device. For far-field or T-wave oversensing, prolongation of the refractory period will also correct the problem. The sensing polarity may be reprogrammed to bipolar if the option is available and the patient has a bipolar lead. In some instances, surgical intervention may be indicated to repair the lead, replace the lead or upgrade to a bipolar system. Loose set screw almost always needs corrective surgery as well as lead dislodgement. Lead fracture, if not complete, can be managed by changing the programming from a bipolar lead to a unipolar, using the functioning lead channel.

2.1.4. Diaphragmatic pacing and extracardiac stimulation

Diaphragmatic stimulation may result from inadvertent right phrenic nerve pacing by the right atrial lead or by direct stimulation of the diaphragm or chest wall muscle by the ventricular lead. Extracardiac stimulation occurs due to poor lead placement and/or high output pacing. Lead

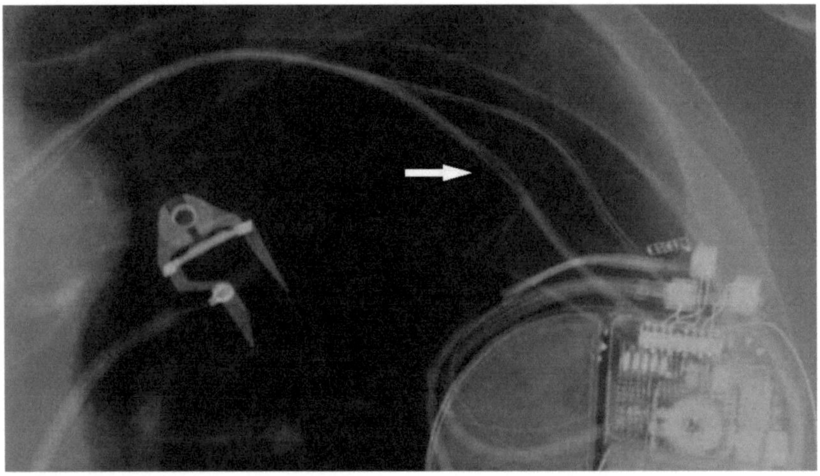

Image 1. Chest radiography demonstrating a lead fracture (arrow) resulting in high lead impedance.

perforation through the myocardial wall may cause extracardiac stimulation [10]. Unipolar pacemakers and leads with failed outer insulation may trigger stimulation of tissue adjacent to the site of the exposed conductor coil.

2.1.4.1. Corrective action

Decrease output if possible while maintaining an adequate safety margin for cardiac capture. Revision of the culprit lead may be required. Reprogram to bipolar polarity if unipolar.

2.1.5. Pacemaker syndrome

Pacemaker syndrome can occur in patients in sinus rhythm who receive a VVI pacing system or in patients with a dual-chamber device if the atrial lead fails to properly capture or sense

Image 2. Chest radiography showing two loose set screws (black arrows) resulting in lead noise and high impedance. After pocket revision and proper reconnection of both lead device and lead parameters normalized.

[11]. Ventricular pacing asynchronous to atrial contraction will limit the atrial contribution to ventricular filling. The resultant decline in cardiac output may cause patient fatigue and discomfort whenever the pacemaker is pacing. The classic example of pacemaker syndrome is caused by retrograde AV-nodal conduction. When the ventricle is paced and contracts, the depolarization impulse travels in a retrograde manner up the His bundle through the AV node towards the atrium. The atrium then contracts while the mitral and tricuspid valves are closed due to simultaneous ventricular contraction. The late atrial contraction causes blood to flow retrograde into the venous system resulting in "cannon A-waves," dyspnea, hypotension, fatigue or even syncope. The surface ECG can give important clues to the correct diagnosis. In many cases, a retrograde inverted P-wave is seen embedded in the T-wave, as a sign of ineffective (as well as detrimental) atrial contraction. Patients with diastolic dysfunction, pericardial disease or loss of ventricular compliance due to hypertension, ischemic heart disease, ventricular hypertrophy or age are more likely to experience pacemaker syndrome.

2.1.5.1. Corrective action

For VVI devices, reduce the pacing rate or program a hysteresis rate to allow more time in sinus rhythm. If device reprogramming fails to resolve the problem, upgrade to a dual-chamber pacemaker is indicated. A malfunctioning atrial lead in a dual-chamber system may either be reprogramed or require surgical correction.

2.1.6. Pacemaker-mediated tachycardia (PMT)

Pacemaker-mediated tachycardia (PMT), also referred to as endless-loop tachycardia or ELT, is an abnormal state caused by the presence of an accessory conducting pathway (the pacemaker) [12]. The mechanism of tachycardia is similar to that seen in patients presenting with the Wolff-Parkinson-White Syndrome. PMT often begins with a premature ventricular beat that is either spontaneous or pacemaker induced (**Figure 14**). The electrical impulse traverses retrograde through the His bundle and AV node to the atrium. The pacemaker will sense the retrograde P-wave if it falls outside of the postventricular atrial refractory period (PVARP). This will trigger an AVI after which the pacemaker will pace the ventricle. This cycle will repeat itself until one of the following occurs: (1) the retrograde P-wave blocks at the level of the AV node, (2) the retrograde P-wave falls within PVARP, (3) a magnet is applied to the pacemaker (disabling sensing) or (4) the device is reprogrammed to a longer PVARP or AV interval. The patient may use standard vagal maneuvers to induce transient AV block, thereby terminating the tachycardia. Though not commonly used for this purpose, adenosine (or any other AV-nodal blocking agent) may be given to terminate the tachycardia. PMT may initiate or restarted if a ventricular-sensed beat precedes an atrial beat. This includes a PVC, premature junctional beat, loss of atrial sensing or capture, and myopotential tracking or inhibition in the atrium. Appropriate programming of the PVARP will prevent PMT such that any retrograde P-wave will fall within this interval and therefore not be sensed by the atrial channel. However, some patients have markedly prolonged AV-nodal conduction and the long PVARP that is necessary to prevent PMT may severely limit the maximum tracking rate of the device due to the resulting long total atrial refractory period (TARP). Most modern pacemakers offer PMT prevention, yet still allow programming a short PVARP. One option automatically extends the PVARP for one cardiac cycle whenever a sensed R-wave is

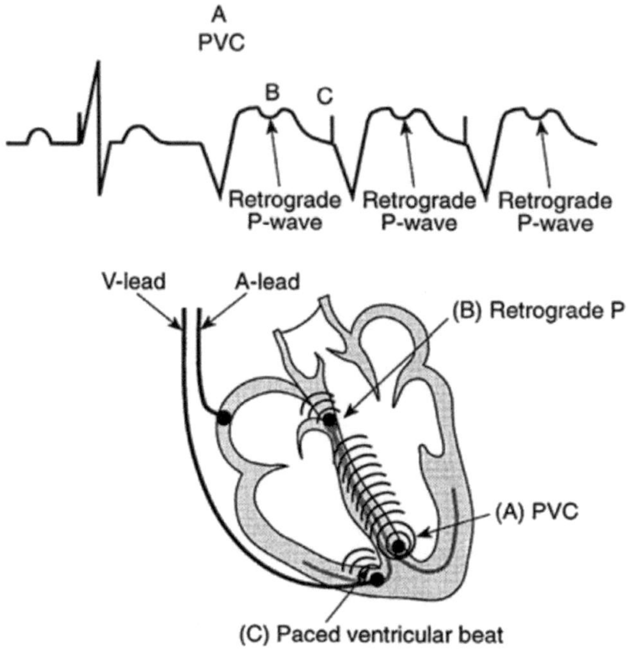

Figure 14. Pacemaker-mediated tachycardia (PMT): a PVC occurs (A) causing the ventricle to contract. The electrical impulse conducts retrograde through the AV node (B) resulting in atrial contraction. The retrograde P-wave is sensed by the pacemaker, which initiates an AV interval (AVI). At the end of the AVI, a pacing stimulus is delivered to the ventricle (C) and the cycle continues.

not preceded by a paced or sensed P-wave (assuming a PVC). An alternative method is to disable atrial sensing after a PVC is detected. This is also known as "DVI on PVC" since no atrial sensing takes place for one cardiac cycle. When first introduced by Pacesetter, it was known as "DDX" (some of these older devices are still in use today). The newest prevention algorithm will force an atrial output when sensing a PVC. Pacing the atrium at the time of a PVC will result in collision of anterograde and retrograde beats in the AV node, thus preventing the onset of PMT. Finally, most current devices provide an automatic termination algorithm if PMT is suspected. When the pacemaker reaches the upper rate (or a separately programmable PMT detection rate) for a specified number of beats, the PVARP is extended for a single cycle or alternatively a DVI cycle is introduced or atrial pacing is delivered, terminating PMT if present.

Figure 15 shows two different scenarios when atrial tachycardia (AT) can be misdiagnosed as pacemaker-mediated tachycardia (PMT).

1. An AT at a rate below the upper tracking limit is sensed on the atrial channel triggering an impulse on the ventricular channel.

2. Pacing in the atrial channel can suppress or terminate AT.

3. Prolonging the PVARP may lead to 2:1 atrioventricular conduction without interrupting the AT.

http://dx.doi.org/10.5772/intechopen.69998

4. In true PMT, ventricular activation causes retrograde atrial activation which is sensed on the atrial channel triggering ventricular depolarization.
5. Pacing in the atrium during PMT interrupts the tachycardia but cannot differentiate PMT from AT (see [2])
6. Prolonging the PVARP will result in termination of PMT with resumption of sinus rhythm, while an underlying AT will conduct to the ventricle at exactly half the tachycardia rate.

In conclusion, prolonging the PVARP is a better method to differentiate AT from PMT and effectively terminate PMT.

2.1.7. Crosstalk

This is a potentially dangerous or lethal problem in patients who are pacemaker dependent [2]. Crosstalk occurs if the ventricular sensing amplifier misinterprets the atrial pacing impulse for an intrinsic ventricular beat. Ventricular output is inhibited and in patients without a ventricular escape rhythm, asystole will occur. On the surface, ECG crosstalk results in paced atrial P-waves without subsequent ventricular output. As a characteristic finding, the atrial pacing interval is equal to the atrial escape interval (AEI), rather than AVI and AEI combined. The shortened pacing interval results because the AVI is terminated prematurely due to the ventricular circuit falsely identifying the atrial pacing pulse for an intrinsic ventricular beat resetting the pacemaker to the next cycle. However, in a device using atrial-based timing, the AVI will be allowed to complete before the next AEI ensues, thus maintaining

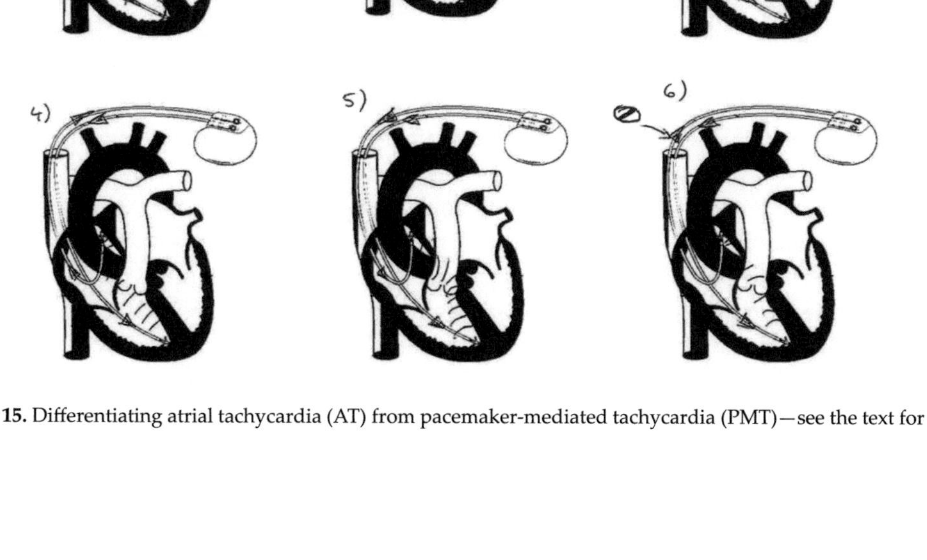

Figure 15. Differentiating atrial tachycardia (AT) from pacemaker-mediated tachycardia (PMT)—see the text for details.

the programmed pacing rate. Crosstalk is more likely to occur if high atrial output pacing is combined with very sensitive settings on the ventricular channel.

Most modern pacemakers are very resistant to crosstalk and certain features can prevent or reduce the effect of crosstalk. "safety pacing," also known as "ventricular safety standby" or "nonphysiologic AV-delay" ensures a brief period of ventricular sensing during the early postatrial output period. This special sensing interval immediately following the ventricular blanking period is known as the "crosstalk-sensing window" (CTW). An event falling into the CTW may be the result of crosstalk or of true ventricular origin. If the ventricular lead senses an event during the CTW, a ventricular pacing output is committed at a short AV-delay (usually 100–120 ms), providing ventricular rate support should crosstalk be present. In the presence of a PVC or other intrinsic beat, use of a short AV-delay ensures that the ventricular output is not delivered during the relative refractory period (vulnerable period) of the T-wave (**Figure 11a**). While this feature will avoid the detrimental effects of crosstalk, the underlying cause needs be identified and corrected as soon as possible.

Figure 16 represents an example of crosstalk: the atrial impulse delivered by the pacemaker is sensed on the ventricular channel resulting in inhibition of a ventricular output. In summary, the management of crosstalk includes:

1. Decreasing sensitivity of the ventricular channel

2. Decreasing output of the atrial channel

3. Activating ventricular safety pacing

4. Increasing the ventricular blanking period

5. Decreasing atrial pulse width

6. If the cause of crosstalk is insulation failure, implantation of a new atrial lead is warranted.

2.2. Defibrillator troubleshooting

Failure of the ICD to deliver a shock during ventricular tachycardia or ventricular fibrillation may result in presyncope, syncope or death. Conversely, inappropriate shock therapy causes patient discomfort, increases health care expenditure due to device clinic visits and/or hospitalization and heightens mortality [13]. Since all commercially available ICDs provide anti-bradycardia pacing their use is subject to the same potential problems as regular pacemakers. In addition, the dedicated bipolar ICD lead is used for tachycardia detection and treatment. In an "integrated bipolar" system, one of the shocking electrodes has the added function of a sensing and pacing anode. The ICD gathers information on the low-voltage impedance of the pacing system and the high-voltage impedance during shock delivery. The ability to evaluate the low- and high-voltage components separately can help the physician localize the site of lead failure. Adding a separate pacing/sensing lead may be a simple solution when only the low-voltage conductor is affected. However, failure of the high-voltage component often requires lead extraction and replacement. In certain circumstances, a second shocking coil may be added without removing the malfunctioning lead. The approach to the patient with suspected ICD malfunction is essentially the same

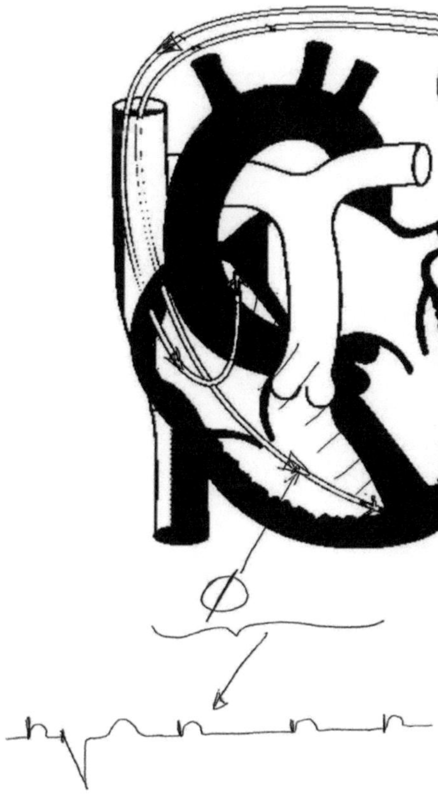

Figure 16. Crosstalk: atrial activation is sensed on the ventricular channel resulting in inhibition of ventricular pacing.

as the approach described for the pacemaker patient. Gathering patient data, understanding the indication for device implant, ICD interrogation, and evaluating the circumstances surrounding the incident in question are all essential. A common clinical scenario is the need to assess whether an ICD shock was appropriately delivered. For ICDs with limited diagnostic capability, elucidating the history surrounding the shock is crucial. The delivery of an appropriate ICD shock is often preceded by palpitations, lightheadedness, dyspnea or syncope. However, even in the absence of aforementioned symptoms, an appropriate ICD shock may have been delivered. Symptomatic hypotension may not ensue if the patient is in a sitting or supine position. Alternatively, the patient may simply not recollect the event due to insufficient brain perfusion or the patient was asleep at the time of the arrhythmic event. Indeed, nocturnal myoclonus is frequently misinterpreted by the patient's spouse as a device discharge. Inappropriate ICD shocks most commonly occur in the setting of AF. In the setting of AF with a ventricular response rate that exceeds the detection rate of the device, the ICD will charge and deliver one or repetitive shocks. Occasionally, the shock will convert AF to sinus rhythm. Dual-coil ICD leads with the proximal coil located within the right atrium are more likely to convert AF to sinus rhythm than single-coil leads. Importantly, these shocks are not the result of device malfunction, but rather due to an undesirable patient-device interaction. The specific categories of device malfunction are noted below.

2.2.1. Failure to shock or deliver anti-tachycardia pacing

Failure of the ICD to deliver anti-tachycardia therapy may be lethal. The reasons for failure to shock are listed as follows [14]:

1. Undersensing
    a. Lead malposition
    b. Lead dislodgment
    c. Lead perforation
    d. Lead fracture
    e. Lead insulation failure
    f. Lead-to-device connector problem
    g. Sensitivity set too low (i.e. insensitive)
    h. Poor electrogram amplitude due to change in myocardial substrate
    i. Myocardial infarction
    j. Drug therapy
    k. Metabolic imbalance
    l. "Fine" ventricular fibrillation
2. Primary circuit failure
3. Battery failure
4. Shock therapy turned off (by programming or magnet)
5. Magnet placed over the device
6. Strong magnetic field present
7. Detection rate set too high
8. Failure to meet additional detection criteria
    a. Rate stability
    b. Sudden onset
    c. Morphology criteria
9. Slowing of tachycardia below detection rate
    a. Substrate changes
    b. Metabolic changes

http://dx.doi.org/10.5772/intechopen.69998

c. Electrolyte changes

d. Drug therapy changes

10. Interaction with permanent pacemaker

Lead failure or programming the rate detection zone too high is the most common reason for failure of the ICD to deliver therapy. The cause for lead failure may be identified on fluoroscopy. As older transvenous ICD leads are substantially thicker than conventional pacing leads, they are exposed to higher forces below the clavicle when using a subclavian vein access. Lead fracture typically affects one of the inner conductors of a coaxial or triaxial lead. Sometimes an intact outer conductor shielding a fractured inner conductor complicates proper diagnosis on fluoroscopy. Fractures can result in two broken ends remaining in intermittent contact. Several fluoroscopic projections may be required to visualize conductor failure and a slightly over-penetrated fluoroscopic image with settings similar to a dedicated thoracic spine view should be used. Fractures and insulation failures are more likely to occur after 1 or more years. If undersensing develops within 30 days of ICD implant, lead malposition, lead dislodgment or lead perforation need to be considered. Rarely, a loose connection between a connector pin and a connector block is the cause for ICD failure. Although ICDs are generally very reliable, a number of alerts have been reported for different models. Circuit failure, software lock-up, and other problems do occur infrequently and proper device interrogation will usually not be possible if any of these situations are present. In some cases, a "system reset" may be able to resolve the problem. In other cases, a software patch downloaded to the device will correct the problem.

Patient noncompliance with routine device clinic follow-up may result in ICD failure due to battery depletion. The ICD may become nonfunctional or lack sufficient power to charge the capacitors to the required voltage for discharge. Most ICDs restrict the time allowed for the capacitor to charge. Should the battery reserve be too low or the capacitor be defective (a common problem in earlier devices), the charge time may exceed the maximum time allowed and the ICD will not deliver a shock.

Occasionally, the rate detection zone is set too high. This may result from inappropriate programming or more commonly initiation of antiarrhythmic drug therapy such as amiodarone or sotalol. Antiarrhythmic drugs may cause slowing of the ventricular tachycardia cycle length below the programmed detection rate [15]. Significant metabolic or electrolyte abnormalities can affect the tachycardia cycle length, but may also alter the signal amplitude resulting in undersensing or failure to detect. Use of additional detection criteria to enhance specificity may delay or prevent appropriate ICD therapy and should be applied cautiously. Tissue injury due to myocardial infarction may lead to significant changes in the intracardiac electrogram and failure to sense.

Asynchronous pacing can be seen if bradycardia backup-pacing is turned on. In the past, many patients requiring pacing support underwent additional pacemaker implantation to prevent early ICD battery depletion from frequent pacing. This is usually of no clinical consequence unless the ICD senses the pacing output delivered by the pacemaker. In a worst-case scenario, the pacemaker may misinterpret ventricular fibrillation for asystole and attempt to pace fibrillating myocardium. If the ICD were falsely interpret the pacing impulse from the pacemaker for a regular Waveforms of ventricular depolarization (QRS) complex, device therapy may be withheld indefinitely. For this reason, special care is exercised if a pacemaker patient undergoes additional ICD implantation or a dedicated pacemaker is indicated in an ICD patient. Be aware that, albeit less likely, oversensing of the atrial pacemaker impulse by the ICD may lead to similar grave consequences.

2.2.1.1. Corrective action

Defibrillator lead-related problems virtually always require surgical correction. Most physicians argue that lead failure requires lead removal due to the large size of the lead and potential interaction with a newly placed lead. A recently implanted ICD lead that has dislodged or demonstrated poor sensing performance may be repositioned if lead integrity can be verified. Immediate device replacement is indicated in the case of battery depletion or if a nonfunctional ICD fails software reset. Simple reprogramming of the ICD will resolve problems related to inappropriate tachycardia detection zones or if too many specificity criteria are applied to diagnose ventricular tachycardia causing delay or failure to deliver appropriate therapy. Interaction with a permanent pacemaker may be eliminated by reprogramming the pacemaker output and pulse width to lower values. Only a bipolar pacemaker should be implanted if an ICD is already present. Furthermore, the pacemaker should be a dedicated bipolar device or allow bipolar pacing as the "power-on-reset" polarity. The latter will prevent reset to unipolar polarity and guarantee pacing in the bipolar mode if power is temporarily interrupted. Since current ICDs integrate full-featured pacing capabilities, a separate pacemaker is rarely indicated. Noise due to lead fracture can cause oversensing with inhibition of output. Acute management includes changing to a unipolar configuration or sensing from a wider antenna, for example, lead tip to right ventricle (RV) coil, until the lead can be replaced.

2.2.2. Failure to convert ventricular arrhythmia

Despite proper detection and appropriate ICD therapy, some arrhythmic episodes may fail to convert to sinus rhythm with potentially lethal consequences for the patient. Below is a list of problems that may prevent restoration of sinus rhythm despite appropriate ICD therapy [15]:

- High defibrillation threshold
- Poor cardiac substrate (fibrosis, scar, etc.)
- Acute myocardial infarction
- Metabolic abnormality
- Electrolyte abnormality
- Drug therapy
- Drug proarrhythmia
- High-voltage lead fracture

http://dx.doi.org/10.5772/intechopen.69998

- High-voltage lead insulation failure
- High-voltage lead migration
- Inappropriate device programming
- Low (inadequate) shock energy
- Ineffective polarity
- Sub-optimal "tilt"
- Ineffective pacing sequence
- Pacemaker polarity switch
- Atrial arrhythmias
- Sinus tachycardia
- "VT Storm"

Changes to the myocardial substrate following successful ICD implantation may result in delayed or unsuccessful antiarrhythmic therapy. Acute myocardial infarction, severe electrolyte or metabolic imbalance or initiation of antiarrhythmic drug therapy may increase the defibrillation threshold. Amiodarone is frequently utilized in patients presenting with life-threatening arrhythmias and may increase the defibrillation threshold. Some patients will require defibrillation threshold testing after amiodarone initiation to verify successful conversion with ICD shock delivery. Other drugs may act proarrhythmic to the effect that the arrhythmia fails to convert or resumes immediately after conversion. Lead fracture or insulation failure will reduce the actual amount of energy delivered to the heart and may impact the delivery of an effective ICD shock. Lead movement may alter the shock vector resulting in suboptimal current flow between anode and cathode.

Programming the shock energy below maximum output will conserve battery life, allow quicker shock delivery, and cause less pain to the patient. However, an insufficient safety margin between defibrillation threshold and applied energy reduces the probability of successful conversion. The shock duration (pulse width) is programmable on some devices and set automatically on others. If set too short or overly long, defibrillation will be unsuccessful. The optimal shock duration varies based on the resistance. The positive and negative phases of the shock wave may be programmable in duration and can significantly affect efficiency of therapy. Furthermore, anti-tachycardia pacing or low-energy shock delivery may accelerate ventricular tachycardia or cause degeneration into ventricular fibrillation.

2.2.2.1. Corrective action

Immediately correct reversible metabolic, drug or electrolyte abnormalities. Lead or device problems will often require surgical revision. Reprogram ICD to a different rate detection zone and/or reassess additional criteria applied for tachycardia recognition. Atrial arrhythmias may require drug therapy, catheter ablation to definitive treatment of the clinical arrhythmia or ablation of the AV node. Appropriate pacemaker selection and programming are mandatory if separate devices are used in the same patient. Strongly consider replacement for a single device.

2.2.3. Inappropriate ICD therapy

Inappropriate ICD shocks are far more common than failure to convert or failure to deliver therapy. Patients may think an ICD shock was delivered inappropriately, while thorough evaluation of telemetry data and stored electrograms confirms proper device therapy. If the ICD shock was determined inappropriate, the triggering event needs to be elucidated and corrected quickly. Repeat ICD shocks are poorly tolerated by the conscious patient because of pain encountered and fear of future episodes. The patient may voice anger and frustration or demand device removal. Although inappropriate shocks are less likely to result in patient death, immediate diagnosis and correction of the underlying cause are warranted. Causes for inappropriate ICD therapy are as follows [16]:

1. Oversensing

    a. Electromagnetic interference
    b. Interaction with another implanted device
    c. Lead fracture
    d. Lead insulation failure
    e. Loose connections
    f. Myopotentials
    g. T-Wave oversensing
    h. Pacing impulse from permanent pacemaker
    i. "Y" adapted biventricular adapters and connectors

2. Detection rate set too low
3. Supraventricular arrhythmias

    a. Paroxysmal supraventricular tachycardia
    b. Atrial fibrillation
    c. Atrial flutter
    d. Sinus tachycardia

Inappropriate shocks are most commonly encountered in the presence of atrial fibrillation. Many patients who undergo ICD implantation demonstrate enlarged hearts predisposing them to atrial tachyarrhythmias. Patients with a history of slow ventricular tachycardia may experience overlap with sinus tachycardia at the lower rate limit of the detection zone. This may occur during exercise, sexual intercourse or emotional stress and result in ICD shock.

Oversensing may lead to inappropriate detection as detailed above. Interactions may result from separate pacemaker and ICD implantation in the same patient. In the presence of a unipolar and some bipolar pacemakers, the ICD may sense the ventricular and/or atrial pacing spike resulting in double-counting of the ventricular rate during VVI pacing or triple-counting of the ventricular rate during DDD pacing. Double-sensing may also be seen with some biventricular devices if the right and left ventricles are wired into the same sensing circuit, for example, when using a "Y" adapter on the pacing lead to connect to a single ventricular connector on the device. It may also be the result of an older ICD design where, despite separate connectors available for the RV and left ventricle (LV) lead, the leads are interconnected within the device and run through a single pace/sense circuit. The net result of both of these configurations is the same, with the RV and LV lead being sensed on the same channel. Double-counting may occur due to the long conduction delay between RV and LV if the patient has a heart rate in excess of the URL, or one of the leads fails to capture.

2.2.3.1. Corrective action

The ICD detection rate should be increased if the sinus rate overlaps with the lower rate limit of the detection zone. Beta-blocker therapy should be initiated or uptitrated to reduce the sinus rate. Furthermore, additional discrimination criteria such as sudden onset, rate stability, and QRS morphology should be activated. Catheter ablation to treat the clinical atrial arrhythmia or ablation of the AV node may be an option in select patients. Interaction between pacemaker and ICD will require reprogramming to a lower output and pulse width, using bipolar polarity or upgrading to an integrated pacemaker and ICD system. The latter is often necessary if double-sensing occurs while using retained older leads or ICD connector designs. In some situations, the pacing lead may require repositioning. Lead failure and connection problems will often require urgent surgical correction. If EMI is detected, the patient should be advised to avoid the source of interference. For some patients, this may involve reassignment of duties at work or even a change in employment. Most ICD malfunctions and pseudo-malfunctions are readily diagnosed after obtaining a careful patient history, use of fluoroscopy, and device interrogation. Unnecessary replacement of the ICD will be avoided and patient safety and comfort assured if competent personnel addresses the device problem in a consistent manner.

3. Conclusion

In order to troubleshoot implantable cardiac devices, the clinician should have a thorough understanding of the underlying physics and signal processing techniques. Device implantation and follow-up requires knowledge of the most common causes for device malfunction. While device reprogramming may offer a permanent solution for some pacemaker or ICD malfunctions, others will require surgical correction as appropriate first-line therapy.

Author details

Sorin Lazar*, Henry Huang and Erik Wissner

*Address all correspondence to: slazar1@uic.edu

Division of Cardiology, Section of Cardiac Electrophysiology, University of Illinois at Chicago, Chicago, IL, USA

References

[1] Lyons RG. Understanding Digital Signal Processing. 2nd ed. Prentice Hall PTR Upper Saddle River, NJ, USA, 2004

[2] Ellenbogen KW, Kay N, Lau CP, Auricchio A. Clinical Cardiac Pacing, Defibrillation and Resynchronization Therapy. Elsevier Radarweg 29, 1043 NX Amsterdam, The Netherlands; 2016

[3] Berold S. Cardiac Pacemakers Step by Step. Blackwell Publishing

[4] Natale A. Handbook of Cardiac Electrophysiology. UK: Informa, 2008

[5] Lloyd MS, El Chami MF, Langberg JJ. Pacing features that mimic malfunction: a review of current programmable and automated device functions that cause confusion in the clinical setting. Journal of Cardiovascular Electrophysiology. 2009;**20**(4):453-460

[6] Roos M, Kobza R, Erne P. Early pacemaker battery depletion caused by a current leak in the output circuitry: rectification not exchange. Pacing and Clinical Electrophysiology. 2007;**30**(5):705-708

[7] Brambatti M, Mathew R, Strang B, Dean J, Goyal A, Hayward JE, et al. Management of patients with implantable cardioverter-defibrillators and pacemakers who require radiation therapy. Heart Rhythm. 2015;**12**(10):2148-2154

[8] Maisel WH, Sweeney MO, Stevenson WG, Ellison KE, Epstein LM. Recalls and safety alerts involving pacemakers and implantable cardioverter-defibrillator generators. The Journal of the American Medical Association. 2001;**286**(7):793-799

[9] Hayes DL, Vlietstra RE. Pacemaker malfunction. Annals of Internal Medicine. 1993;**119**(8): 828-835

[10] Laborderie J, Barandon L, Ploux S, Deplagne A, Mokrani B, Reuter S, et al. Management of subacute and delayed right ventricular perforation with a pacing or an implantable cardioverter-defibrillator lead. The American Journal of Cardiology. 2008;**102**(10):1352-1355

[11] Link MS, Hellkamp AS, Estes NA 3rd, Orav EJ, Ellenbogen KA, Ibrahim B, et al. High incidence of pacemaker syndrome in patients with sinus node dysfunction treated with ventricular-based pacing in the mode selection trial (MOST). Journal of the American College of Cardiology. 2004;**43**(11):2066-2071

[12] Ausubel K, Gabry MD, Klementowicz PT, Furman S. Pacemaker-mediated endless loop tachycardia at rates below the upper rate limit. The American Journal of Cardiology. 1988;**61**(6):465-467

[13] Poole JE, Johnson GW, Hellkamp AS, Anderson J, Callans DJ, Raitt MH, et al. Prognostic importance of defibrillator shocks in patients with heart failure. The New England Journal of Medicine. 2008;**359**(10):1009-1017

[14] Swerdlow CD, Asirvatham SJ, Ellenbogen KA, Friedman PA. Troubleshooting implanted cardioverter defibrillator sensing problems I. Circulation: Arrhythmia and Electrophysiology. 2014;**7**(6):1237-1261

[15] Swerdlow CD, Friedman PA. Advanced ICD troubleshooting: Part II. Pacing and Clinical Electrophysiology. 2006;**29**(1):70-96

[16] Israel CW. How to avoid inappropriate therapy. Current Opinion in Cardiology. 2008; **23**(1):65-71

Chapter 6

ICD Electrograms in Patients with Brugada Syndrome

Cismaru Gabriel, Serban Schiau, Gabriel Gusetu,
Lucian Muresan, Mihai Puiu, Radu Rosu,
Dana Pop and Dumitru Zdrenghea

Additional information is available at the end of the chapter

http://dx.doi.org/10.5772/intechopen.70145

Abstract

In patients with Brugada syndrome, implantable cardioverter-defibrillator (ICD) is the only demonstrated treatment that prevents sudden cardiac death. The progress in ICD technology improved the diagnosis and efficacy of implantable devices in the management and treatment of ventricular tachycardia (VT) and ventricular fibrillation (VF). Recording of electrical events just before and after a delivered or aborted ICD therapy permits a more accurate characterization of the rhythm but also provides information on the electrical events preceding the arrhythmia. This chapter aims to gain insight into the mechanism of initiation and termination of spontaneous VF by analyzing intracardiac electrograms (IEGM) in Brugada patients implanted with ICDs. It has two parts: **(1) update on ICD electrograms in Brugada syndrome patients**, where we review the medical literature on ICD electrograms and their use for detecting electrical manifestations of Brugada syndrome, and **(2) examples of ICD electrograms,** from our own database of patients affected by Brugada syndrome.

Keywords: Brugada syndrome, ICD, defibrillation, ventricular fibrillation, premature ventricular contractions, electrophysiological study

1. Introduction

Brugada syndrome is a clinical syndrome associated with ventricular tachycardia (VT) and ventricular fibrillation (VF), in patients who have no structural heart disease. ECG is the most useful tool for the diagnosis and shows right bundle branch block with ST elevation in right precordial leads. Due to the high recurrence rate of ventricular fibrillation, an implantable cardioverter-defibrillator (ICD) is the accepted mode of treatment and it improves the long-term prognosis.

Clinical studies suggest that spontaneous episodes of VF are induced by PVCs originating at the level of right ventricular outflow tract (RVOT). Abnormal electrophysiological features are present in this zone, with fragmented, low amplitude, late potentials. Programed ventricular stimulation at the level of RVOT increases the chance of VF induction compared to RV apex.

The progress in ICD technology improved the diagnosis and treatment efficacy of implantable devices in the management of VT and VF in Brugada syndrome. Recording of electrical events before and after a delivered or aborted ICD therapy permits not only a more accurate characterization of the rhythm but also provides information on the electrical events preceding the arrhythmia.

2. Mode of onset of ventricular fibrillation in Brugada syndrome

In Brugada syndrome, VF episodes can be preceded by PVCs or start suddenly without a preceding premature ventricular contractions (PVC). This classification assumes distinct electrophysiological mechanism for the two types of VF. Although very few PVCs are observed on Holter monitoring, in Brugada syndrome PVCs tend to occur more frequently before the initiation of VF, as well as ST segment elevation in precordial leads [1]. The mechanism that explains the association of the two phenomena is the marked shortening of the action potential in the RVOT which gives the ST elevation, and phase 2 reentry responsible for PVC firing from the same area with short action potential, which initiates VF [2, 3]. Kofune et al. were able to identify the substrate of the Brugada syndrome by high-resolution electroanatomical mapping. In patients with Brugada syndrome, they found that only the right ventricle is affected, the left being spared, and only a small area within the RVOT is responsible for the syndrome. At this level, they found low-voltage potential with fractionated electrograms. The conduction abnormality from the RVOT gives the final phenotypic expression of right precordial ST segment elevation [4]. Previous studies of Antzelevitch et al. demonstrated that at cellular level the action potential dome propagates from the normal epicardial sites to the epicardial site without dome leading to phase 2 reentry. As the reentry fails to propagate to the endocardium, it leads to closely coupled ventricular premature beats [5]. Specific triggers can lead to heterogeneous repolarization: fever or after exercise when the body temperature rises, and specific medication like: ajmaline, flecainide, and propafenone.

In the study of Kakishita et al., frequent PVCs before the onset of VF were recorded in 67% of the patients. The morphology of preceding PVC electrogram (far-field and near-field) was identical to the PVC that initiated VF. Additionally, different VF episodes seen in the same patient were initiated by the same PVC morphology. The rest of 33% of patients had episodes of VF without preceding PVCs.

A long-short sequence is very unlikely to initiate VF in Brugada syndrome and pause-dependent VF is very rare [6].

http://dx.doi.org/10.5772/intechopen.70145

3. Coupling interval of the VF initiating PVC

It is well known that PVCs occurring near the peak of the T-wave (ventricular vulnerable period) may lead to ventricular fibrillation. However, in Brugada syndrome, the onset of PVCs inducing VF are close to the end of the T-wave. Kakishita et al. found a coupling interval of 388 ms for the PVC initiating VF in patients with Brugada syndrome. Kasanuki et al found a value of > 300 ms coupling interval for the PVC inducing VF. Spontaneous VF is provoked by a single, long >300 ms coupled PVC. Induced VF can be provoked by multiple extrastimuli with shorter coupling interval < 200 ms for VF induced during electrophysiological study [7].

4. Ventricular fibrillation interval (VF interval)

For long time, physicians thought that the amplitude of VF waves ("fine" or "coarse") is suggestive of defibrillation success, but Murakawa et al. demonstrated on dogs [8] that shorter ventricular fibrillation intervals are associated with higher energies for internal defibrillation. VF interval is a parameter that can be measured using the ICD electrograms. Kerber et al. [9] reported that slower polymorphic VT with cycle length >200 ms needs less energy for defibrillation than VF with cycle length of less than 200 ms. Cismaru et al. studied VF cycle length in patients with Brugada syndrome, induced VF during electrophysiology study, and showed that a longer cycle length that progressively increases is a sign of self-terminating VF [10] (**Figures 1** and **2**).

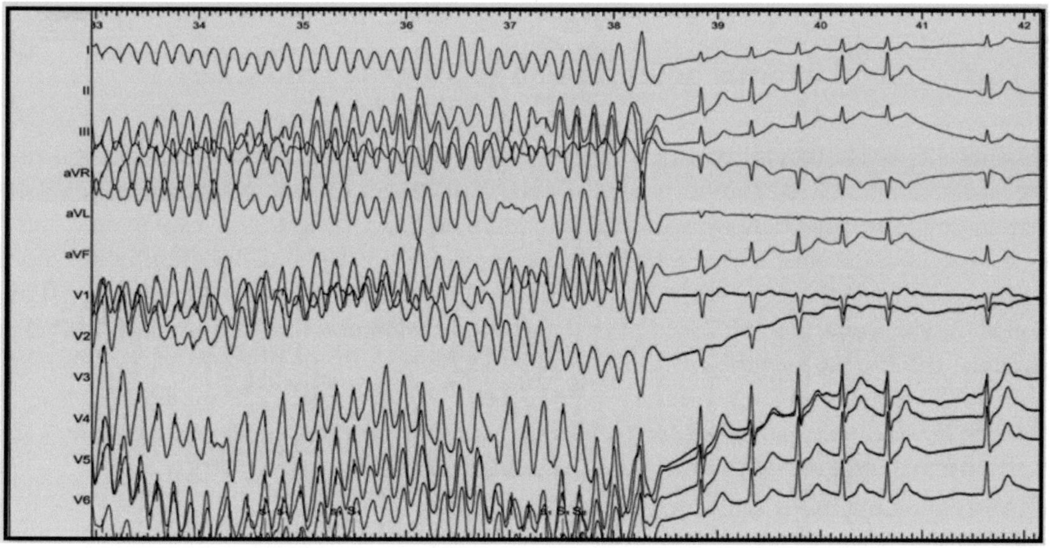

Figure 1. Patient with Brugada syndrome and polymorphic VT induction during electrophysiology study. VT stops spontaneously without any defibrillation.

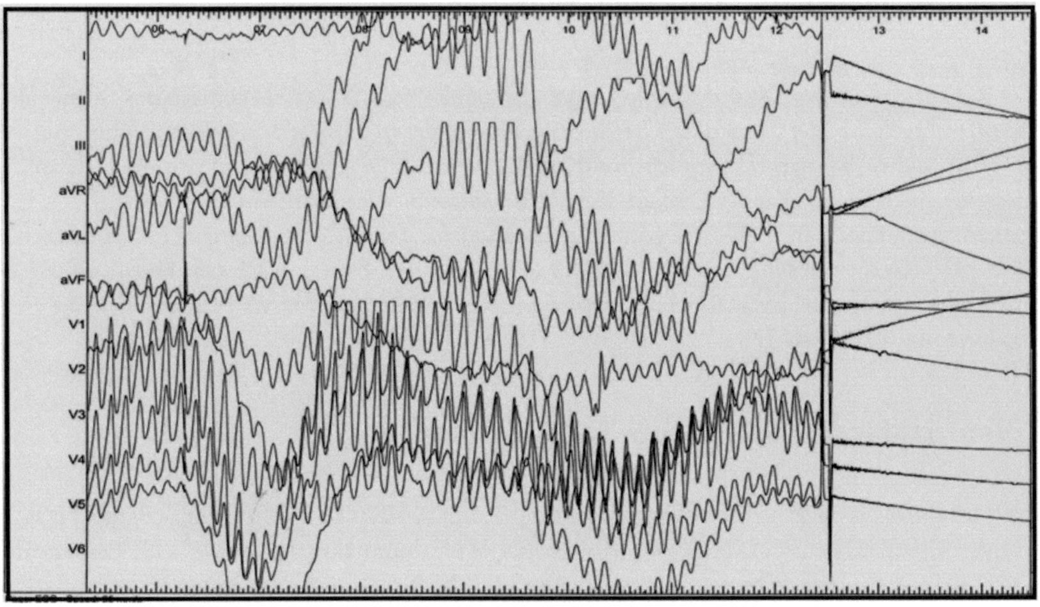

Figure 2. Patient with Brugada syndrome and ventricular fibrillation induction during electrophysiology study. Please note the short VF interval. VF stops after external defibrillation.

Hiratsuka et al. demonstrated that symptomatic patients with Brugada syndrome have significant shorter VF cycle length than asymptomatic patients. The difference is probably given by a different electrophysiological substrate between the two groups [11].

5. Unsuccessful internal defibrillation in Brugada syndrome

Patients with Brugada syndrome have higher rates of unsuccessful internal defibrillation after the implantation of ICD. The study of Watanabe et al. [12] examined the incidence of VF not responding to internal defibrillation and found an incidence of 18%. One explanation could be the origin of the electrical abnormality at the level of RVOT [13] with defibrillation shock delivered between the right ventricular apex and left subclavicular can. Alternative explanation is the short effective refractory period and short ventricular fibrillation interval (FVI) in patients with Brugada syndrome.

6. Intracardiac electrograms (IEGM) compared to morphological changes of an ECG during provocative tests

Probst et al. [14] compared the surface ECG with the intracardiac electrograms (IEGM) from internal defibrillator during an ajmaline test in patients with Brugada syndrome. The ECG morphology changed after ajmaline injection with ST elevation and negative T-waves. The IEGM showed different morphological changes: ST deviation changes with negative T-wave

http://dx.doi.org/10.5772/intechopen.70145

changes. The changes are in contrast with morphological changes from patients without Brugada syndrome where IEGM correlates to ST segment deviation on ECG. In countries where ajmaline is not available, procainamide can be used for the provocative test.

In the case report of Moore and Kaye, a change of the intracardiac electrogram after an internal defibrillation was compatible with a type 1 Brugada pattern and disappeared 1 min after the electrical shock [15, 16].

7. T-wave alternans in patients with Brugada syndrome

T-wave alternans is the ECG manifestation of action potential repolarization alternans. Beat-to-beat alternation of ventricular action potential in both duration and amplitude reflects the risk of ventricular tachycardia and ventricular fibrillation [16]. T wave alternance (TWA) from ICD electrograms are concordant with TWA from the surface ECG because they measure the same alternans phenomenon [17] (**Figure 3**).

Tada et al. described a patient with Brugada syndrome that presented TWA after administration of a sodium channel blocker (cibenzoline) [18]. Ohkubo et al. also described TWA in a patient with Brugada syndrome after class 1 antiarrhythmic drug (pilsicainide). TWA persisted for 15 min and was followed by microvolt TWA [19].

Tada and colleagues [20] investigated the association between ventricular tachycardia and fibrillation with TWA induced by intravenous pilsicainide (sodium channel blocker). Pilsicainide provoked visible TWA in 17 of 77 Brugada patients. Those with TWA experienced a significantly higher incidence of spontaneous VF (52.9 vs. 8.3%) than those without TWA.

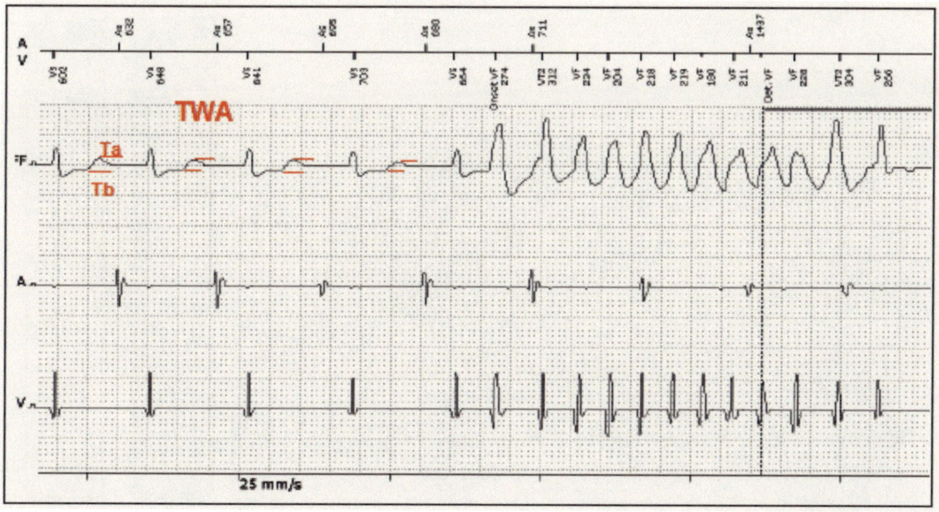

Figure 3. Method for determination of TWA: the amplitude for each T-wave is calculated as the maximum minus the minimum value (horizontal red lines). The difference between the amplitude of the first beat and second beat of each pair is calculated using the formula: TWA = $[(Ta–Tb)_1+(Ta–Tb)_2+\ldots(Ta–Tb)_x]/x$.

8. Use of stored ICD electrograms for catheter ablation of ventricular fibrillation in Brugada syndrome

Stored electrograms can be used for catheter ablation of ventricular fibrillation. Both far-field EGM and near-field EGM are used [21]. First, the EGM that initiates ventricular fibrillation should be captured. This is used as a template for subsequent pacemapping (**Figure 4**). Information regarding the morphology and timing of the EGM are used to search for the best correlation during pacemap. Both spontaneous QRS complex morphology and far-field ICD morphology are used for comparison with the paced morphology. Timing between far-field and near-field ICD electrograms is also used for the template when comparing with the paced beat.

Pacemapping is attempted at the level of RVOT with real-time recording from the ICD electrogram. Both morphology and timing are used to delineate the zone with the best match and that zone will be a target for ablation. The study of Almendral et al. [22] showed spatial resolution of 2 cm^2 for best match with electrogram morphology and timing. The same resolution was confirmed by Lowery et al. in patients with different types of ventricular fibrillation [21].

Substrate epicardial mapping is initiated in sinus rhythm to identify dense scar <0.5 V and border zone between 0.5–1.5 V. Abnormal electrograms consist in low amplitude–wide duration of >80 ms, with multiple or delayed components outside the end of the surface ECG QRS. The same RVOT zone is remapped after IV flecainide to determine increase in abnormal electrogram area after infusion. Catheter ablation targets the complete elimination of the substrate inside the low-voltage areas [23].

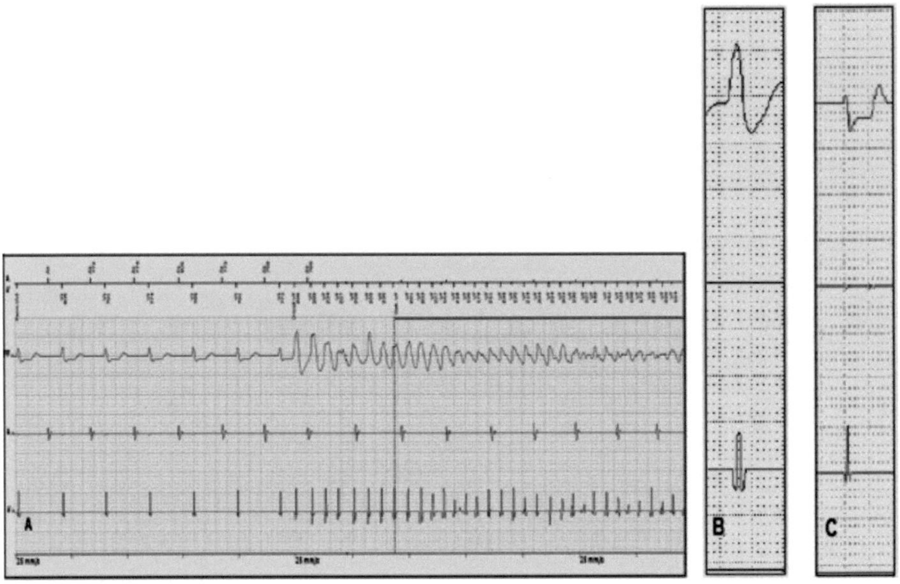

Figure 4. Example of pacemapping of a trigger arising from the RVOT in a patient with Brugada syndrome. Panel A corresponds to the recorded spontaneous PVC inducing VF (A). Panels B and C show near- and far-field electrograms with a bad correlation between the spontaneous RVOT (B) and paced electrogram (C).

9. Examples of ICD electrograms

We present electrograms from our cardiology department in patients with Brugada syndrome:

- Coupling interval of the PVC initiating ventricular fibrillation (**Figures 5** and **6**).
- Safe terminating ventricular tachycardia (**Figures 7** and **8**).
- Ventricular fibrillation terminated by an electrical shock (**Figure 9**).

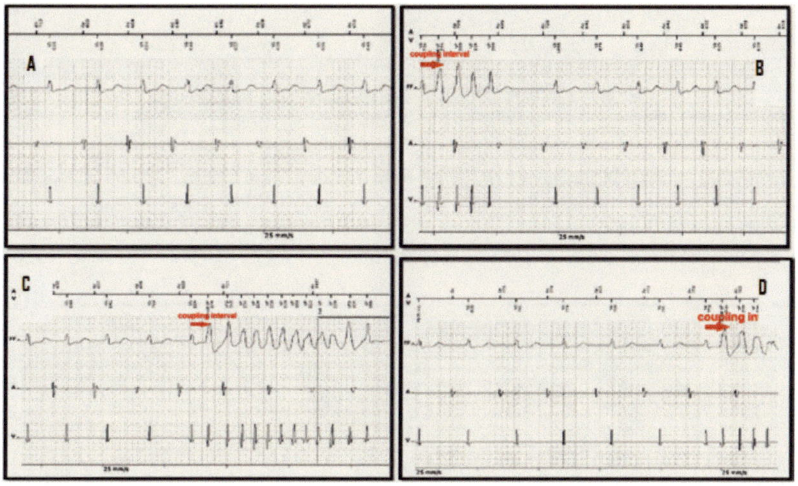

Figure 5. The same coupling interval 330 ms and the same PVC morphology at the initiation of nonsustained VT in a patient with Brugada syndrome. (A) without PVCs; (B) PVC inducing NSVT; (C) same PVC inducing NSVT; (D) same PVC inducing NSVT.

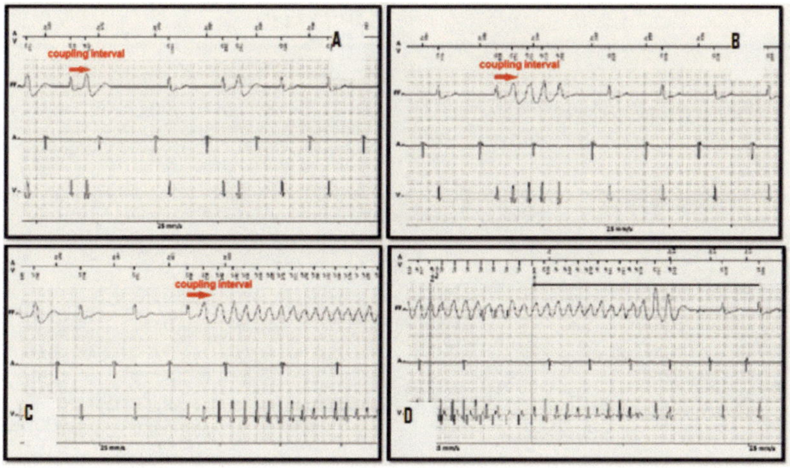

Figure 6. The same coupling interval 322 ms and same morphology at the initiation of nonsustained VT in a patient with Brugada syndrome. (A) PVCs with ventricular trigeminism; (B) same PVC inducing NSVT; (C) same PVC inducing (D) self-terminating VF.

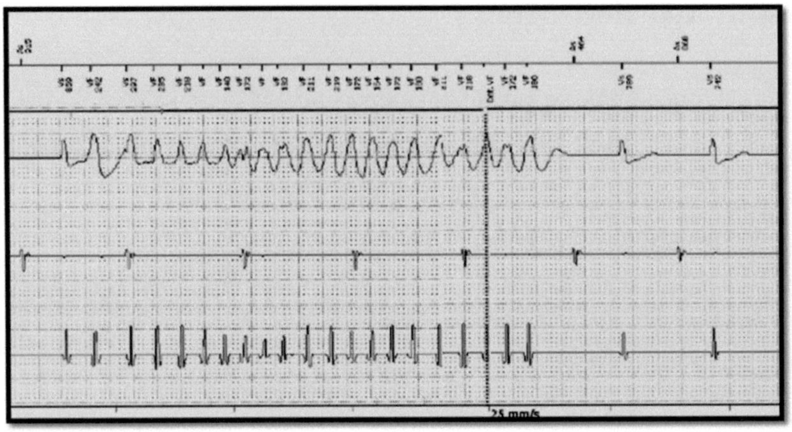

Figure 7. Self-terminating ventricular tachycardia. Please note the long cycle length. Upper electrogram is the far-field ventricular IEGM; in the middle of the strip atrial IEGM; at bottom near-field ventricular IEGM.

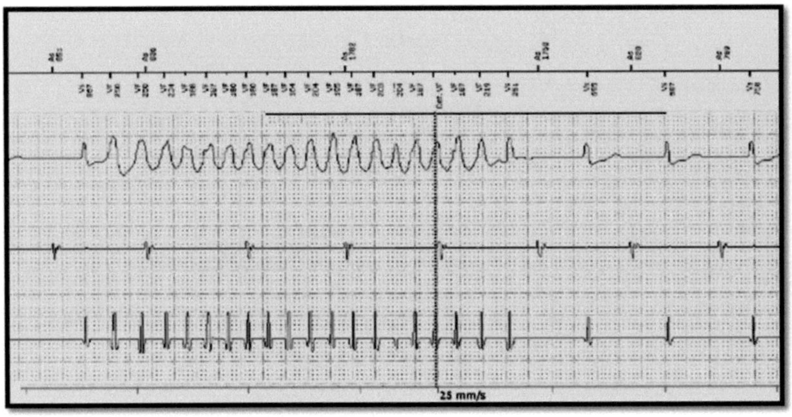

Figure 8. Self-terminating (or nonsustained) ventricular tachycardia. Please note the long cycle length.

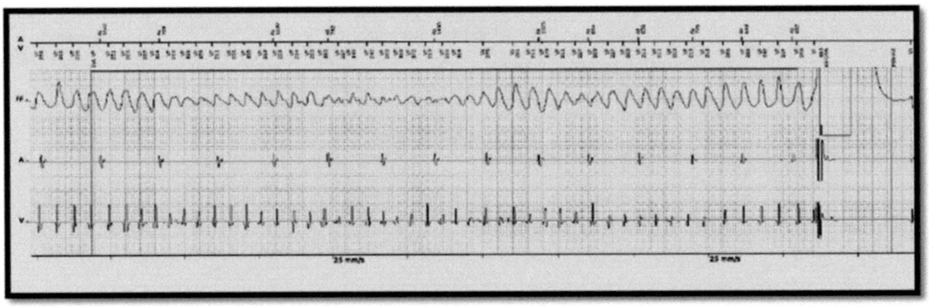

Figure 9. Ventricular fibrillation terminated with an external shock. Please note the short VF interval.

10. Conclusion

Analysis of intracardiac electrograms during episodes of ventricular arrhythmias is effective for clarifying the mechanism of the episode. Many spontaneous episodes of VF are preceded by frequent PVCs. The coupling interval usually is long and reaches the end of the T-wave. Ventricular fibrillation interval is short and may be responsible for failure of internal defibrillation. Longer VF interval values predict spontaneous termination of VF. A catheter ablation technique was described for catheter ablation of PVCs initiating VF in Brugada syndrome and uses the stored IEGMs as template for pacemapping.

Author details

Cismaru Gabriel*, Serban Schiau, Gabriel Gusetu, Lucian Muresan, Mihai Puiu, Radu Rosu, Dana Pop and Dumitru Zdrenghea

*Address all correspondence to: gabi_cismaru@yahoo.com

Cardiology-Rehabilitation, Internal Medicine Department, Iuliu Hatieganu University of Medicine and Pharmacy, Cluj-Napoca, Romania

References

[1] Kasanuki H, Ohnishi S, Ohtuka M, et al. Idiopathic ventricular fibrillation induced with vagal activity in patients without obvious heart disease. Circulation. 1997;**95**:2277-2285

[2] Antzelevith C, Sicouri S, Lukas A, et al. Clinical implications of electrical heterogeneity in the heart: The electrophysiology and pharmacology of epicardial M and endocardial cell. In: Podrid PJ, Kowey PR, editors. Cardiac Arrhythmia: Mechanism, Diagnosis and Management. Baltimore: Williams and Wilkins; 1995. pp. 88-107

[3] Lukas A, Antzelevitch C. Differences in the electrophysiological response of canine ventricular and endocardium to ischemia: Role of the transient outward current. Circulation. 1993;**88**:2903-2915

[4] Kofune M, Watanabe I, Okhubo K, et al. Clarifying the Arrhythmogenic substrate for Brugada Syndrome. Electroanatomic mapping study of the right ventricle. Int Heart J. 2011;**52**:290-294

[5] Antzelehich C, Fish JM, Diego JM. Cellular Mechanisms Underlying the Brugada Syndrome: From Bench to Bedside. Malden MA: Blackwell-Futura; 2005. pp. 52-77

[6] Kakishita M, Kurita T, Matsuo K, Taguchi A, Suyama K, Shimizu W, Aihara N, Kamakura S, Yamamoto F, Kobayashi J, Kosakai Y, Ohe T. Mode of onset of ventricular fibrillation

in patients with Brugada syndrome detected by implantable cardioverter defibrillator therapy. Journal of the American College of Cardiology. 2000;**36**:1646-1653

[7] Eckardt L, Kirkhhof P, Schulze-Bahr E, et al. Electrophysiologic investigation in Brugada syndrome. Yield of programmed ventricular stimulation at two ventricular sites, with up to three premature beats. European Heart Journal. 2002;**23**:1394-1401

[8] Murakawa Y, Yamashita T, Kanese Y, Sezaki K, Omata M. Is ventricular fibrillation interval an indicator of electrical defibrillation threshold? Pacing and Clinical Electrophysiology. 1999;**22**:302-306

[9] Kerber RE, Kienzle MG, Olhansky B, et al. Ventricular tachycardia rate and morphology determine energy and current requirements for transthoracic cardioversion. Circulation. 1992;**85**:158-163

[10] Cismaru G, Brembilla-Perot B, Pauriah M, Zinzius PY, Sellal JM, Schwartz J, Sadoul N. Cycle length characteristics differentiating sustained from self-terminating ventricular fibrillation in Brugada syndrome. Europace. 2013;**15**:1313-1319

[11] Hiratsuka A, Shimizu A, Ueyama T, Yoshiga Y, Doi M, Ohmiya T, Yoshida M, Fukuda M, Matsuzaki M. Characteristics of induced ventricular fibrillation cycle length in symptomatic Brugada syndrome patients. Circulation Journal.2012;**76**:624-633

[12] Watanabe H, Chinushi M, Sugiura H, Washizuka T, Komura S, Hosaka Y, Furushima H, Hayashi J, Aizawa Y. Unsuccessful internal defibrillation in Brugada syndrome: Focus on refractoriness and ventricular fibrillation cycle length. Journal of Cardiovascular Electrophysiology. 2005;**16**:262-266

[13] Morita H, Fukushima-Kusano K, Nagase S, Takenaka-Morita S, Nishii N, Kakishita M, Nakamura K, Emori T, Matsubara H, Ohe T. Site-specific arrhythmogenesis in patients with Brugada syndrome. Journal of Cardiovascular Electrophysiology. 2003;**14**:373-379

[14] Probst V, Sacher F, Derval N, Gourraud JB, Mabo P, Medkour F, Le Marec H, Gill J. Correlation of intracardiac electrogram with surface electrocardiogram in Brugada syndrome patients. Europace. 2014;**16**:908-913

[15] Moore PT, Kaye GC. Possible late diagnosis of the Brugada syndrome in a patient presenting with a primary cardiac arrest. Europace. 2015;**17**:1839

[16] Pastore JM, Girouard SD, Laurita KR, et al. Mechanism linking T-wave alternans to the genesis of cardiac fibrillation. Circulation. 1999;**99**:1385-1394

[17] Paz O, Zhou X, Gillberg J, et al. Detection of T-wave alternans using an implantable cardioverter-defibrillator. Heart Rhythm. 2006;**3**:791-797

[18] Tada H, Nogami A, Shimizu W, Naito S, Nakatsugawa M, Oshima S, Taniguchi K. ST segment and T wave alternans in a patient with Brugada syndrome. Pacing and Clinical Electrophysiology. 2000;**23**:413-415

[19] Ohkubo K, Watanabe I, Okumura Y, Yamada T, Masaki R, Kofune T, Oshikawa N, Kasamaki Y, Saito S, Ozawa Y, Kanmatsue K. Intravenous administration of class I anti-arrhythmic drug induced T wave alternans in an asymptomatic Brugada syndrome patient. Pacing and Clinical Electrophysiology. 2003;**26**:1900-1903

[20] Tada T, Kusano KF, Nagase S, Banba K, Miura D, Nishii N, et al. Clinical significance of macroscopic T-wave alternans after sodium channel blocker administration in patients with Brugada syndrome. Journal of Cardiovascular Electrophysiology. 2008;**19**:56-61

[21] Lowery CM, Tzou WS, Aleong RG, Nguyen DT, Varosy PD, Katz DF, Hath RR, Schuller JL, Lewkowiez L, Sauer WH. Use of stored implanted cardiac defibrillator electrograms in catheter ablation of ventricular fibrillation. Pacing and Clinical Electrophysiology. 2013;**36**:76-85

[22] Almendral J, Atienza F, Everss E, Castilla L, Gonzales-Torecilla E, Ormaetxe J, Arenal A, et al. Implantable defibrillator electrograms and origin of left ventricular impulses: An analysis of regionalization ability and visual spatial resolution. Journal of Cardiovascular Electrophysiology. 2012;**23**:506-514

[23] Brugada J, Pappone C, Berruezo A, Vicedomini G, et al. Brugada syndrome phenotype elimination by epicardial substrate ablation. Circulation Arrhythmia and Electrophysiology. 2015;**8**:1373-1381

Chapter 7

A Review of ICD Anti-Tachycardia Therapy Programming with Generic Programming for Primary and Secondary Prevention

Fariha Sadiq Ali and Usama Boles

Additional information is available at the end of the chapter

http://dx.doi.org/10.5772/intechopen.69999

Abstract

Intracardiac defibrillator plays a pivotal role in preventing sudden cardiac death; however, inappropriate shock delivery remains an important source of morbidity and mortality. Advancements in device technology along with various shock reduction strategies play a key role in reducing inappropriate and unnecessary shocks. Anti-tachycardia pacing (ATP) is the first-line therapy prior to shock delivery. Several trials have validated the efficacy of ATP for both slow and fast ventricular tachycardia without significant increase in occurrence of arrhythmia-related syncope. In addition, trials also support that therapy for non-sustained tachycardia can be prevented by higher programmed zones and prolonged intervals to detect without higher risk of syncope. With this perspective, authors employ a customized programming for both primary and secondary prevention to reduce inappropriate therapies or unnecessary therapies, in particular, progression to shock but allow for spontaneous termination at slower ventricular tachycardia rates. The programming was instituted at the time of device implantation or at follow up.

Keywords: intracardiac defibrillator, anti-tachycardia pacing, inappropriate therapies, shock, customized programming, ICD programming, ICD therapies, reducing ICD therapies, ICD templates

1. Introduction

Implantable cardioverter-defibrillator (ICD) remains the main therapeutic option in reducing sudden cardiac death (SCD). Several randomized trials and registries have shown that ICD extends survival in patients with severe left ventricular function and mild-to-moderate heart failure [1–4]. The shocks delivered whether appropriate, inappropriate or unnecessary remain an important source of mortality and morbidity from proarrhythmic potential, heart failure, painful delivery of shock causing significant anxiety, depression and post-traumatic stress disorder [5–11].

Inappropriate ICD shocks are those delivered for a condition other than true ventricular arrhythmias, which most commonly include supraventricular arrhythmias with rapid rates, mechanical failure of ICD lead/system like lead conductor fracture resulting in noise detection and non-mechanical issues such as T-wave over sensing resulting in double-counting [3]. Unnecessary or potentially avoidable shocks are those where the ventricular tachycardia (VT) was to terminate spontaneously or could have been interrupted by appropriately timed pacing stimuli.

Table 1 lists the major clinical trials and registries reporting the incidence of inappropriate shocks. We review some of the trials here.

The anti-arrhythmics versus implantable defibrillators (AVID) was a multi-centre trial which patients were randomized to receive ICD or anti-arrhythmic drug therapy; 492 patients were randomized to receive an ICD over a follow-up period of 22 ± 12 months. Inappropriate shocks in this cohort were due to supraventricular tachycardia in 18% and 3% were due to ICD malfunction or inappropriate sensing [12].

The Pain FREE Rx II trial was a prospective randomized control trial consisting of 634 patients with a mean follow up of 11 ± 3 months. All patients received ICDs and were randomized to anti-tachycardia pacing versus shock only programming [13]. There were 4230 spontaneous episodes retrieved from all implanted ICDs, 1837 had complete electrogram data and were included in the analysis. Of these, 491 episodes (27%) were determined to be inappropriately detected supraventricular tachycardia (SVT), and 4 (0.2%) were non-physiological artifact. Sweeny et al. performed a subgroup analysis of the PainFree trial and showed that the proportion of true ventricular detections that resulted in shocks was similar between primary and secondary prevention groups (40% versus 32%, respectively) [14]. The proportion of inappropriate ventricular detections due to SVT that resulted in shocks was also similar between primary and secondary prevention groups (44% versus 42%, respectively).

MIRACLE ICD was a prospective, randomized double-blind trial of 978 patients with a mean 10-month follow-up [15]. This trial evaluated the safety and efficacy of cardiac resynchronization combined defibrillator therapy (CRT-D) versus ICD only therapy in both primary and secondary prevention patients. The reported incidence of inappropriate shocks was 30% in primary prevention patients and 14% in secondary prevention patients.

In the Multicenter Automatic Defibrillator Implantation Trial II (MADIT-II), inappropriate shocks constituted 31.2% (184/590) of the total shock episodes [16]. The most common triggers were atrial fibrillation (44%) and supraventricular tachycardia (36%) with improper discrimination by the ICD device, followed by abnormal sensing (20%). The majority of inappropriate ICD therapy episodes were delivered for rhythms below or equal to 200 bpm; the mean ventricular rate triggering inappropriate shock for atrial fibrillation (AF) or SVT was 174 ± 22 bpm. Patients with inappropriate ICD shocks showed a significantly higher mortality during the follow-up (HR = 2.29, 95% CI: 1.11–4.71, p = 0.02) than patients with

Clinical trial	AVID [12]	PainFREE [13]	MIRACLE ICD [15]	MADIT II [16]	SCD-Heft [17]	ALTITUDE ICD [18]	ALTITUDE CRT-D [18]	Leidin [19]
Patient no.	449	582	978	719	811	39,396	29,904	1544
Follow up, months	22	11	10	20	46	28	28	41
Single/dual	Single/dual	Single/dual	Single/dual	Single/dual	Single	Single/dual	Single/dual	Single/dual
Primary/secondary	Secondary	Primary/ secondary	Primary/ secondary	Primary	Primary	Primary/ secondary	Primary/ secondary	Primary/ secondary
Inappropriate Rx, %	21	15	14–30*	12	17	16	17	18
Inappropriate Rx, (HR, 95% CI, *p*)	n.a	n.a	n.a	2.29 (1.11–4.71) 0.02	1.98 (1.29–3.05) 0.002	1.84 (1.30–2.61)	1.60 (1.15–2.23)	1.60 (1.10–2.30) $p = 0.01$
Appropriate Rx, %	68	33	23–31**	21	23	23	23	n.a
Appropriate Rx, (HR, 95% CI, *p*)	n.a	n.a	n.a	3.36 (2.04–5.55) <0.01	5.68 (3.97–8.12) <0.001	2.05 (1.55–2.71)	2.51 (2.01–3.14)	1.60 (1.20–2.10) <0.01
ATP (yes/no)	Yes	Yes	Yes	Yes	No	Yes	Yes	Yes
Outcome measure	n.a	n.a	n.a	Mortality	Mortality	Mortality	Mortality	Mortality

*14% in secondary prevention and 30% in primary prevention.

**23% in primary prevention and 31% in secondary prevention.

Table 1. List of ICD clinical trials and registries with frequency of appropriate and inappropriate therapy and outcome.

appropriate ICD shocks (HR = 3.36, 95% CI: 2.04–5.55, $p < 0.01$). This demonstrated that all shocks, although demonstrated to save lives, also have a detrimental effect and lead to heart failure deterioration and eventual mortality.

Similar data could be extrapolated from the sudden cardiac death in heart failure trial (SCD-HeFT) [17]. In this trial, 2521 patients with primary prevention indication and with mild-to-moderate heart failure were randomized in equal proportions to receive placebo, amiodarone or a single-chamber ICD programmed to shock-only mode. Follow-up was for an average of 46 months. In 811 patients assigned to the ICD arm, the rate of inappropriate shocks was 17% as compared to 22.4% appropriate shocks during a 46-month follow-up. Patients with an inappropriate ICD therapy had a twofold increase in the risk of all-cause mortality (HR = 1.98, 95% CI: 1.29–3.05, $p = 0.002$).

The results from the randomized trials were confirmed in larger registries. The ALTura Impact on the Treatment of Abdominal Aortic Aneurysms Using a Novel D-stent EVAR Design (ALTITUDE) registry involved 39,396 ICD patients and 29,904 patients implanted CRTDs. Patients were implanted for both primary and secondary indications [18]. The 1-year incidence of inappropriate shocks was 8% and 6% and at 5 years increased to 16% and 17% for ICD and CRT-D patients, respectively. The two most common reasons for shock were atrial flutter/atrial fibrillation and sinus tachycardia or supraventricular arrhythmia. Inappropriate shock was due to noise, artifact or over sensing in 3% of the episodes.

The Leiden group published a large scale study in 1544 ICD patients and reported an 18% incidence of inappropriate ICD therapy over 41 months of follow-up. This study also confirmed the increased risk of death for both inappropriate and appropriate ICD therapy (HR1.60 for both, $p = 0.01$ for inappropriate; $p < 0.01$ for appropriate ICD therapy) [19].

2. Possible mechanism of increased risk of death with ICD shocks

It may be hypothesized that there is a direct mechanical or hemodynamic effect of the inappropriate ICD therapies themselves or that some of the inappropriate ICD therapies lead to fatal pro-arrhythmia due to an increase in sympathetic discharge, which in turn leads to rate-related changes in ventricular refractoriness and worsened myocardial ischemia [20].

It is likely that it is not the inappropriate shock *per se* that is detrimental, but the sequelae that hastens the adverse clinical outcome.

It has been suggested that high shock fields are associated with changes in electrophysiological properties of the heart and can be the primary source of activation wave fronts that may give rise to idioventricular rhythms after the shock and perhaps may even perpetuate ventricular fibrillation [21]. The cellular injury from intra-cardiac shock delivery whether it be appropriate or not is reflected in a rise in cardiac troponin I [22]. Though the result may be a rescue from acute ventricular arrhythmia, studies have shown a relationship with increased mortality and morbidity from progression to heart failure as a consequence of the myocardial stunning [5–11].

Minimizing the need for shock delivery overall will, therefore, ultimately prevent the downstream complications.

3. Shock reducing strategies

There have been several technological advancements to improve ICD therapy delivery and to avoid inappropriate and unnecessary ICD therapies. The shock reduction programming strategies may be divided into the following categories:

- Optimizing ventricular tachyarrhythmia discrimination by applying advanced detection algorithms in all therapy zones.
- Delaying onset of anti-tachycardia therapies either by prolonged detection intervals or setting higher tachycardia detection limits.
- Using anti-tachycardia pacing (ATP) as first-line therapy whenever possible prior to shock delivery.

4. Clinical evidence and the rationale to support ATP therapy

Monomorphic VT can be interrupted when an appropriately timed pacing stimulus is delivered into the excitable gap of a re-entrant circuit where a collision with the orthodromic wave front results in termination of the tachycardia.

An alternative explanation is that the paced stimuli result in myocardial depolarization during the relative refractory period. This pre-excites the preceding wave front, thereby altering myocardial excitability and extinguishing the propagation re-entrant VT [23].

The duration of the excitable gap and the conduction time from the pacing stimulus site to the re-entrant circuit are the main factors influencing penetration of the excitable gap and termination of the arrhythmia [24].

Ventricular conduction time is influenced by anatomic and functional barriers as well as the influence of the sympathetic nervous system [25]. The efficacy of the ATP is improved with adequate beta blockade and is not adversely influenced by other anti-arrhythmic drugs as is the case with defibrillation thresholds [26].

5. Customized programming

Several trials have validated the efficacy of ATP in terminating slower cycle length of VT.

The Pain FREE Rx II trial was the first trial that extended the use of ATP for fast VT (FVT) with heart rates of 188–250 beats/min. This study also used longer intervals to detect VT as compared to the previous conventional programming (**Figure 1**) [13, 27]. The result was that 73% of FVT episodes were successfully terminated by the ATP.

It also showed that FVT made up 76% of all ventricular arrhythmias that would have conventionally been treated by shock alone according to conventional ICD programming.

Acceleration of FVT occurred in patients programmed to receive ATP as well as those in the shock only group: 4/273 monomorphic VT episodes (2%) in the ATP arm versus 2/145 (1%) in the shock arm. There were also three episodes of syncope during treatment for FVT (ATP, $n = 2$; shock, $n = 1$). This study, therefore, established the safety and efficacy of ATP for both slow and FVT as first-line therapy in ICDs with a non-significant occurrence or difference in arrhythmia-related syncope in either therapy arm.

The next stage in the evolution of device therapy programming was to defer treatment (VT detection) till absolutely necessary. In this regard, the Primary Prevention Parameters Evaluation (PREPARE) trial (**Figure 2**) [28] evaluated a prolonged detection interval duration of 30/40 ventricular beats and an increased tachycardia detection interval (TDI) of 182 beats/min. Supraventricular detection discrimination algorithms and ATP were also optimized in this programming strategy. Arrhythmic syncope was only 1.6% in the test programming strategy. All-cause mortality in the PREPARE study group was also relatively low (Kaplan-Meier estimated 12-month mortality of 4.9%). Thus, the overall safety behind the rationale of this programming was acceptable.

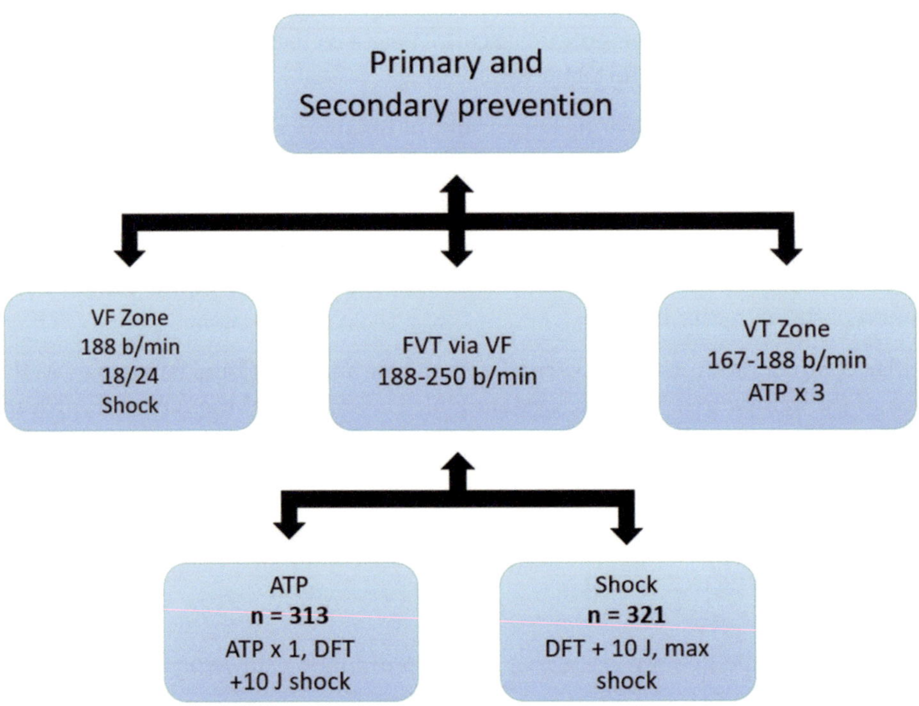

Figure 1. Programming strategy of experimental and control arm in Pain FREE Rx II trial.

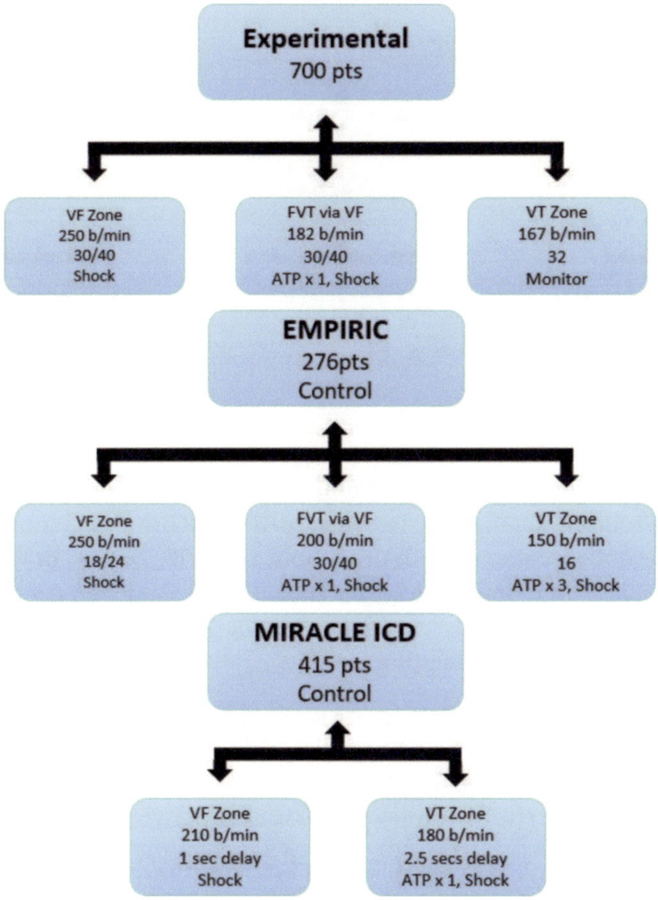

Figure 2. Programming strategy of experimental arm in PREPARE trial with controls from EMPIRIC and MIRACLE ICD patients.

The multicenter automatic defibrillator implantation trial–reduce inappropriate therapy (MADIT-RIT) trial compared three arms: (a) conventional ICD detection of VT with a (b) prolonged detection interval and (c) a higher tachycardia detection interval (**Figure 3**) [29].

The results validated the safety of both the active test arms. There was a 79% reduction in the incidence of therapy in the high-rate group than in the conventional therapy group and delayed therapy (longer detection interval programming) was associated with a 76% reduction in overall therapy delivery. Mortality was reduced by 55% in the high-rate group (p = 0.01) and by 44% in the delayed-therapy group (p = 0.06). Despite withholding therapies till absolutely needed, there was a mortality improvement in these active programming options.

The incidence of syncope was similar between the groups and was not clinically significant: high rate strategy and delayed therapy versus conventional arm (p = 0.39, p = 0.80).

Both delayed therapy and higher rate programming were shown to be safe and efficacious.

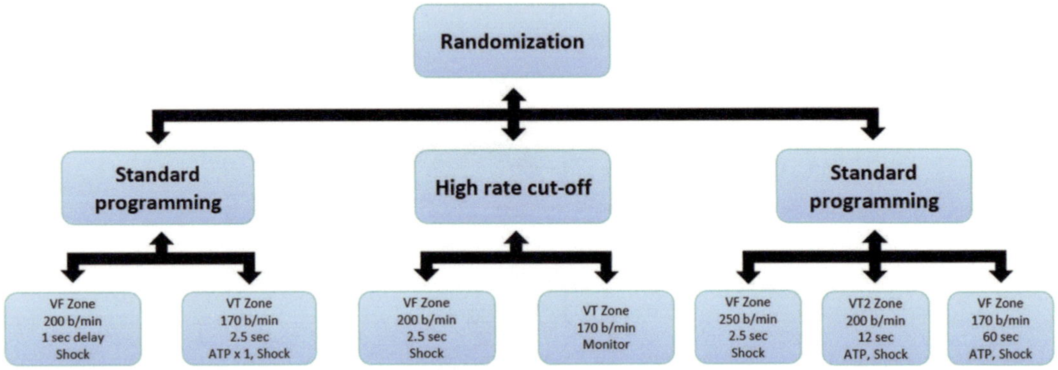

Figure 3. Programming strategy of MADIT-RIT patients.

The ADVANCE III (Avoid Delivering Therapies for Nonsustained Arrhythmias in ICD Patients III) [30] reinforced the findings from the MADIT-RIT trial and included both primary and secondary prevention patients, with or without atrial fibrillation, in whom single-, dual- and triple-chamber ICD were implanted [30]. Thus, this randomized control trial applied an extended detection interval strategy to a heterogeneous cohort of ICD recipients and more likely to resemble a real world setting (**Figure 4**).

This delayed arrhythmia detection strategy resulted in a reduction in the combined end point of all ICD therapies (ATPs and shocks) with 346 delivered therapies (42 therapies per 100 person-years) in test group (extended-detection interval) versus 557 in the control group (standard-detection interval) (67 therapies per 100 person-years); $p < 0.001$.

The incidence of arrhythmic syncope was low in both groups and did not differ significantly with rates of 3.1 versus 1.9 per 100 patient-years ($p = 0.220$ in the extended detection and standard detection groups, respectively). The syncopal episodes were not associated with any additional adverse outcomes. The mortality rates were 5.5 versus 6.3 per 100 patient-years ($p = 0.50$) in extended detection and standard detection, respectively. Both were low and comparable to what was reported in the MADIT-RIT trial.

Similarly the PROVIDE (Programming Implantable Cardioverter Defibrillators in Patients with Primary Prevention Indication to Prolong Time to First Shock) trial was a programming strategy with combination of higher detection rates, prolonged detection intervals, optimized SVT discriminators and empiric ATP therapy compared to conventional parameters in patients receiving ICDs for primary prevention (**Figure 5**) [31]. The primary end point was time to first shock delivery. The median time to first shock was significantly longer at 13.1 months in experimental group versus 7.8 months in the control group. In addition, the 2-year shock rate was 12.4% in the experimental group compared to 19.4% in the control group. An overall reduction in both appropriate and inappropriate shock and ATP was observed. The decrease in ICD therapies was associated with a 30% relative reduction in all-cause mortality.

The incidence of arrhythmic syncope was not significantly different between the two groups with overall incidence of 1.7% over 2 years of follow-up.

With this perspective, we can summarize the overall current trends in ICD programming:

1. Higher zone thresholds
2. Prolonged detection duration or detection intervals
3. Use of advanced discriminators in all zones
4. Use of tiered therapies with ATP as first line therapy before shock delivery.

The aim of these strategies is to reduce inappropriate therapies (ITS) particularly progression to shock and not to over treat ventricular arrhythmias but to allow for spontaneous termination at ventricular rates that are safe to do so.

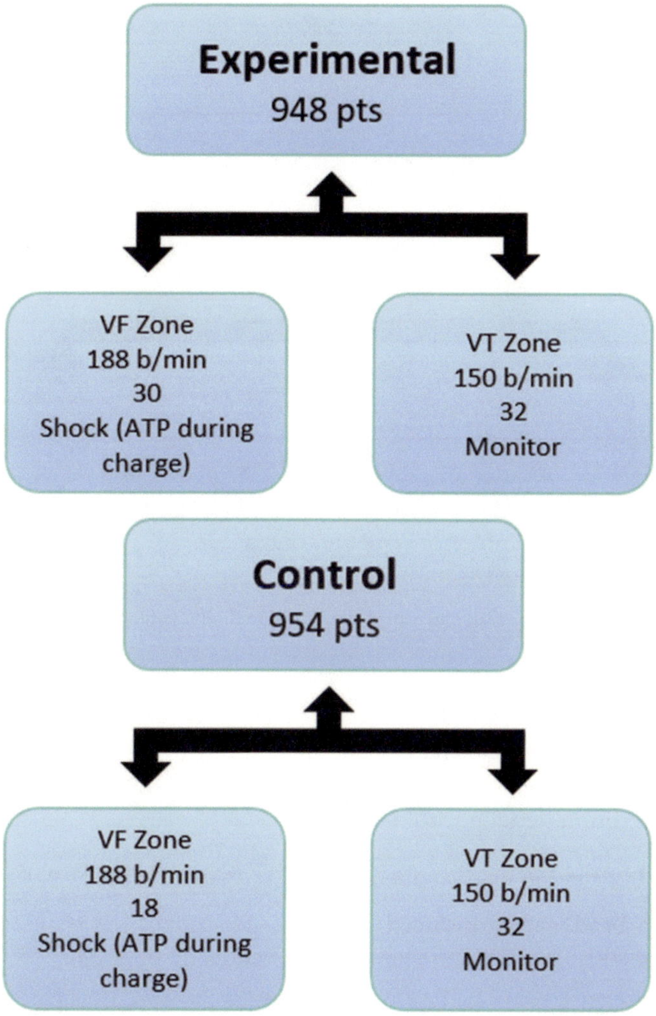

Figure 4. Programming strategy in ADVANCE III trial.

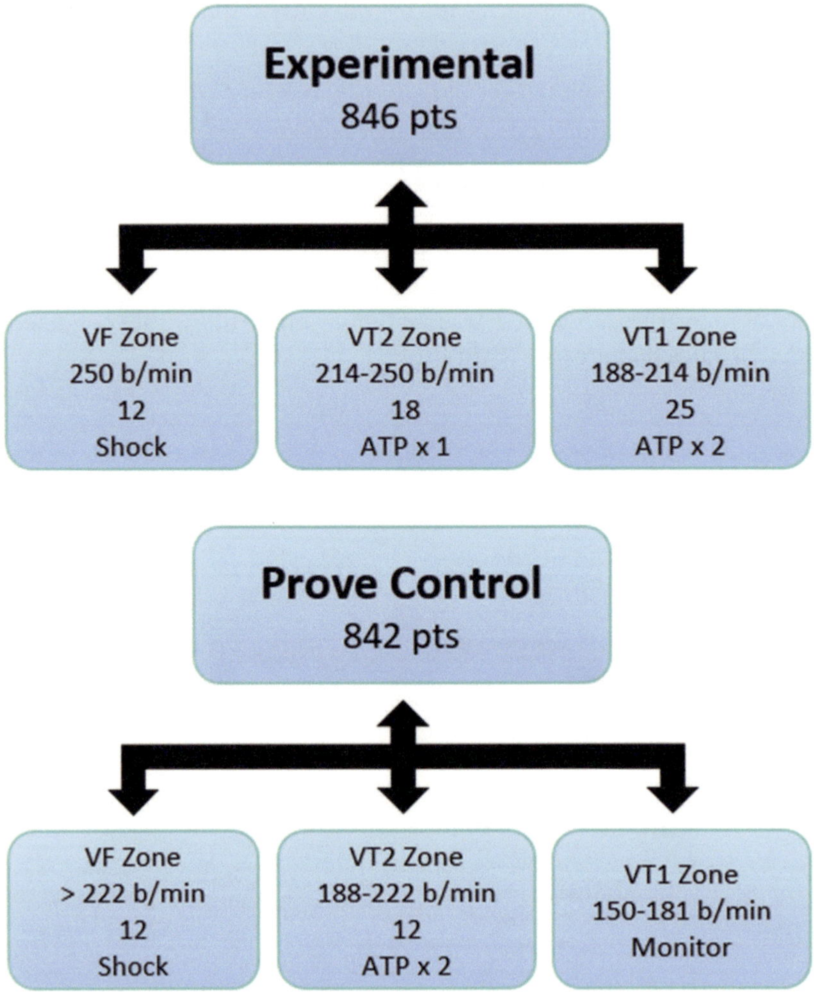

Figure 5. Programming strategy of experimental arm in PROVIDE trial with control population from the PROVE trial.

There has been no data to suggest that implanting dual chamber ICDs is more advantageous in ventricular arrhythmia over single chamber devices in any of the studies we have mentioned. However, there are some practical reasons where one may choose to implant an atrial lead as well to enhance discrimination algorithms [32].

- In patients who require pacing for bradycardia, AV sequential pacing would be preferable.
- In patients with bradycardia-induced or pause-dependent ventricular tachyarrhythmia (such as patients with long QT syndrome and torsades de pointes).
- In patients with documented history of paroxysmal atrial arrhythmias (atrial EGMS will help distinguish the chamber of onset of the tachycardia).

http://dx.doi.org/10.5772/intechopen.69999

- In patients with hypertrophic cardiomyopathy as they are prone to atrial arrhythmias but may also require pacing.

With this in mind, we employ the following customized ICD programming (**Tables 2** and **3**) for both primary and secondary prevention of SCD in our patients.

	Medtronic	**St. Jude medical**	**Biotronik**	**Boston scientific**	**Sorin**
VF (VF + FVT) rate in bpm	230–240	250	250	220	200–240
NID	30	30	12/16	2.5 s initial duration	6 cycles
Therapy	ATP during charge	ATP during charge	ATP: Burst 1	ATP: Burst 1	ATP: Burst 1
	Shock × 6	Shock × 6	Shock × 6	Shock × 6	Shock × 6
VT2 (FVT via VF) CL	250	200	200	200	200
NID	30	30	28 (RD-14)	10 s initial duration	6 cycles
Therapy	ATP: Burst 1	ATP: Burst 1	ATP: Burst 1	ATP: Burst 1	ATP: Burst 1
	Shock × 5	Shocks × 4	Shocks × 5	Shocks × 5	Shocks × 5
VT1 CL in bpm	171	171	171	170	170
NID	28	30	30 (RD-16)	30 s initial duration	12 cycles
Therapy	ATP: Burst 1 + Burst 2	ATP: Burst 1 + Burst 2	ATP: Burst 1 + Burst 2	ATP: Burst 1 + Burst 2	ATP: Burst 1 + Burst 2
	Shocks × 4	Shocks × 3	Shocks × 4	Shocks × 4	Shocks × 4
Monitor CL in bpm	150				150
NID	32				12 cycles
Therapy	None				None
ATP programming					
	Medtronic	St. Jude	Biotronik	Boston	Sorin
Burst 1	8/88/3	8/88/3	8/85/3	8/88/3	8/85/3
Burst 2	8/84/3	8/84/3	8/85/3	8/84/3	8/85/3
Ramp	8/91	8/91	8/90	8/91	8/90

Time out: OFF (Boston Scientific); ATP smart mode: OFF (Medtronic); progressive therapy: ON (Medtronic >2 active zone); ATP optimization: ON (Biotronik); upper rate ATP cut off 260 beats/min (St. Jude); readaptive: ON (St. Jude); Ramp OFF unless specified.

NID: Numbers of interval to detect.

Table 2. Suggested customized ICD programming strategy proposed by the authors for primary prevention.

	Medtronic	St. Jude medical	Biotronik	Boston Scientific	Sorin
VF (VF + FVT) rate in bpm	200	250	250	220	200–240
NID	30	30	12/16	2.5 s initial duration	6 cycles
Therapy	ATP during charge	ATP during charge	ATP: 1 Burst	ATP: Burst 1	
	Shock × 6	Shock × 6	Shock × 6	Shock × 6	Shock × 6
VT2 (FVT via VF) rate in bpm	250	200	200	200	200
NID	30	30	28 (RD-14)	10 s initial duration	6 cycles
Therapy	ATP: Burst 1	ATP: Burst 1	ATP: 1 Burst	ATP: Burst 1	ATP: Burst 1
	Shock × 5	Shocks × 4	Shocks × 5	Shocks × 5	Shocks × 5
VT1 rate in bpm	171/VT-20	171/VT-20	171/VT-20	170/VT-20	170/VT-20
NID	28	30	30 (RD-16)	30 s initial duration	12 cycles
Therapy	ATP: Burst 1 + Burst 2	ATP: Burst 1 + Burst 2	ATP: Burst 1 + Burst 2	ATP: Burst 1 + Burst 2	ATP: Burst 1 + Burst 2
	Shocks ×4	Shocks ×3	Shocks ×4	Shocks ×4	Shocks ×4
Monitor rate in bpm	150/VT-30				150/VT-30
NID	32				12 cycles
Therapy	None				None
ATP programming					
	Medtronic	St. Jude	Biotronik	Boston	Sorin
Burst 1	8/88/3	8/88/3	8/85/3	8/88/3	8/85/3
Burst 2	8/84/3	8/84/3	8/85/3	8/84/3	8/85/3
Ramp	8/91	8/91	8/90	8/91	8/90

Time out: OFF (Boston Scientific); ATP smart mode: OFF (Medtronic); progressive therapy: ON (Medtronic >2 active zone); ATP optimization: ON (Biotronik); upper rate ATP cut off 260 beats/min (St. Jude); readaptive: ON (St. Jude); Ramp OFF unless specified.

Table 3. Suggested customized ICD programming strategy proposed by the authors for secondary prevention.

The programming is instituted at the time of device implantation and refined (if needed) at follow-up in the device clinic.

The programming covers all manufacturers' ICDs that we commonly implant. The custom sets are preloaded onto our programmers, thus minimizing the need for tedious reprogramming and only need to be refined if the case warrants this.

In doing so, the work flow both in the implant suite and at the follow-up device visit is facilitated and the programming can be delegated to our allied professional nurses and cardiac technicians.

6. Conclusion

With the complexity and sophistication of ICD algorithms, the programming of these cardiac devices has become a discipline and challenge in its own right. We have found that it has been difficult to maintain predictability and consistency in the programming of ICDs in our centre, hence a need arose to develop a programming template. This was derived from current trends in programming and is mentioned here in an extensive review of the literature. There is an obvious limitation in which each of the studies has been manufacturer specific. We have tried to identify the principles on which the programming was based and then developed a generic template. This was however still done with due consultation with the manufacturers to ensure applicability and safety with the specific algorithms. There have also been very few studies that deal with programming of secondary prevention of ICDs. We have strived to maintain a compromise between all manufacturers to reach a consensus on programming for primary prevention of ICDs.

Author details

Fariha Sadiq Ali[1]* and Usama Boles[2]

*Address all correspondence to: docham77@hotmail.com

1 Department of Cardiology, Tabba Heart Institute, Karachi, Pakistan

2 Letterkenny University Hospital, Letterkenny, Ireland

References

[1] Moss AJ, Zareba W, Hall WJ, et al. Multicenter automatic defibrillator implantation trial II investigators. Prophylactic implantation of a defibrillator in patients with myocardial infarction and reduced ejection fraction. The New England Journal of Medicine. 2002;**346**:877-883

[2] Bardy GH, Lee KL, Mark DB, et al. Amiodarone or an implantable cardioverter-defibrillator for congestive heart failure. The New England Journal of Medicine. 2005;**352**:225-237

[3] Kadish A, Dyer A, Daubert JP, et al. Prophylactic defibrillator implantation in patients with non-ischemic dilated cardiomyopathy. New England Journal of Medicine. 2004;**350**:2151-2158

[4] A comparison of antiarrhythmic-drug therapy with implantable defibrillators in patients resuscitated from near-fatal ventricular arrhythmias. The Antiarrhythmics versus Implantable Defibrillators (AVID) Investigators. The New England Journal of Medicine. 1997;**337**:1576-1583

[5] Sood N, Ruwald AC, Solomon S, et al. Association between myocardial substrate, implantable cardioverter defibrillator shocks and mortality in MADIT-CRT. European Heart Journal. 2014;**35**:106-115

[6] Powell BD, Saxon LA, Boehmer JP, et al. Survival after shock therapy in implantable cardioverter-defibrillator and cardiac resynchronization therapy-defibrillator recipients according to rhythm shocked. The ALTITUDE survival by rhythm study. Journal of the American College of Cardiology. 2013;**62**:1647-1649

[7] Sweeny MO, Sherfesee L, DeGroot PJ, Wathen MS, Wilkoff BL. Differences in electrical therapy type for ventricular arrhythmias on mortality in implantable cardioverter-defibrillator patients. Heart Rhythm. 2010;**7**:353-360

[8] Poole Je, Johnson GW, Hellkamp AS, et al. Prognostic importance of defibrillator shocks in patients with heart failure. The New England Journal of Medicine. 2008;**4**:1009-1017

[9] Sears SF, Todaro JF, Lewis TS, Sotile W, Conti JB. Examining the psychosocial impact of implantable cardioverter defibrillators: A literature review. Clinical Cardiology. 1999;**22**:481-489

[10] Sears SF, Matchett M, Conti JB. Effective management of ICD patient psychosocial issues and patient critical events. Journal of Cardiovascular Electrophysiology. 2009;**20**:1297-1304

[11] Magyar-Russell G, Thombs BD, Cai J X, Baveja T, Kuhl EA, Singh PP, Montenegro Braga Barroso M, Arthurs E, Roseman M, Amin N, Marine JE, Ziegelstein RC. The prevalence of anxiety and depression in adults with implantable cardioverter defibrillators systematic review. Journal of Psychosomatic Research. 2011;**71**:223-231

[12] Klein RC, Raitt MH, Wilkoff BL, Beckman KJ, Coromilas J, Wyse DG, et al. Analysis of implantable cardioverter defibrillator therapy in the antiarrhythmics versus implantable defibrillators (AVID) trial. Journal of Cardiovascular Electrophysiology. 2003;**14**:940-948

[13] Wathen MS, DeGroot PJ, Sweeney MO, Stark AJ, Otterness MF, Adkisson WO, et al. Pain FREE Rx II Investigators. Prospective randomized multicenter trial of empirical anti tachycardia pacing versus shocks for spontaneous rapid ventricular tachycardia in patients with implantable cardioverter-defibrillators: Pacing fast ventricular tachycardia reduces shock therapies (Pain FREE Rx II) trial results. Circulation. 2004;**110**(17):2591-2596

[14] Sweeney MO, Wathen MS, Volosin K, Abdalla I, DeGroot PJ, Otterness MF, Stark AJ. Appropriate and inappropriate ventricular therapies, quality of life, and mortality among primary and secondary prevention implantable cardioverter defibrillator patients: Results from the pacing fast VT reduces shock therapies (Pain FREE Rx II) trial. Circulation. 2005;**111**(22):2898-2905

[15] Young JB, Abraham WT, Smith AL, Leon AR, Lieberman R, Wilkoff B, et al. Combined cardiac resynchronization and implantable cardioversion defibrillation in advanced chronic heart failure: The miracle ICD trial. JAMA. 2003;**289**:2685-2694

[16] Daubert JP, ZarebaW, CannomDS, McNitt S, RoseroSZ, Wang P, et al. Inappropriate implantable cardioverter-defibrillator shocks in MADIT II: Frequency, mechanisms, predictors, and survival impact. Journal of the American College of Cardiology. 2008;**51**:1357-1365

[17] Poole JE, Johnson GW, Hellkamp AS, Anderson J, Callans DJ, Raitt MH, et al. Prognostic importance of defibrillator shocks in patients with heart failure. The New England Journal of Medicine. 2008;**359**:1009-1017

[18] Saxon LA, Hayes DL, Gilliam FR, Heidenreich PA, Day J, Seth M, et al. Long-term outcome after ICD and CRT implantation and influence of remote device follow-up: The altitude survival study. Circulation. 2010;**122**:2359-2367

[19] van Rees JB, Borleffs CJ, de Bie MK, Stijnen T, van Erven L, Bax JJ, et al. Inappropriate implantable cardioverter-defibrillator shocks: Incidence, predictors, and impact on mortality. Journal of the American College of Cardiology. 2011;**57**:556-562

[20] Pinski SL, Fahy GJ. The proarrhythmic potential of implantable cardioverter-defibrillators. Circulation 1995;**92**:1651-1664

[21] Yabe S, Smith WM, Daubert JP, Wolf PD, Rollins DL, Ideker RE. Conduction disturbances caused by high current density electric fields. Circulation Research. 1990;**66**(5):1190-1203

[22] Hurst TM, Hinrichs M, Breidenbach C, Katz N, Waldecker B. Detection of myocardial injury during transvenous implantation of automatic cardioverter-defibrillators. Journal of the American College of Cardiology. 1999;**34**(2):402-408

[23] Sweeney MO. Antitachycardia pacing for ventricular tachycardia using implantable cardioverter defibrillators. PACE. 2004;**27**:1292-1305. 18

[24] Josephson ME, Almendral JM, Buxton AE, Marchlinski FE. Mechanisms of ventricular tachycardia. Circulation. 1987;**75**:41-47

[25] Fisher JD. Ventricular tachycardia: Practical and provocative electrophysiology. Circulation. 1978;**58**:1000-1001

[26] Jimenez-Candil J, Hernandez J, Martin A, Ruiz-Olgado M, Herrero J, Ledesma C, Morinigo J, Martin-Luengo C. Influence of beta-blocker therapy on anti-tachycardia pacing effectiveness for Monomorphic ventricular tachycardia occurring in implantable cardioverter-defibrillator patients: A dose dependent effect. Europace. 2010;**12**:1231-1238

[27] Wathen MS, Sweeney MO, DeGroot PJ, et al. Shock reduction using anti tachycardia pacing for spontaneous rapid ventricular tachycardia in patients with coronary artery disease. Circulation. 2001;**104**:796-801

[28] Wilkoff BL, Williamson BD, Stern RS, Moore SL, Lu F, Lee SW, et al. PREPARE study investigators. Strategic programming of detection and therapy parameters in implantable

cardioverter-defibrillators reduces shocks in primary prevention patients: Results from the PREPARE (Primary Prevention Parameters Evaluation) study. Journal of the American College of Cardiology. 2008;**52**(7):541-550

[29] Moss AJ, Schuger C, Beck CA, Brown MW, Cannom DS, Daubert JP, et al. MADIT-RIT trial investigators. Reduction in inappropriate therapy and mortality through ICD programming. The New England Journal of Medicine. 2012;**367**(24):2275-2283

[30] Gasparini M, Proclemer A, Klersy C, Kloppe A, Lunati M, Ferrer JB, et al. Effect of long-detection interval vs standard-detection interval for implantable cardioverter-defibrillators on anti-tachycardia pacing and shock delivery: The ADVANCE III randomized clinical trial. JAMA. 2013;**309**(18):1903-1911

[31] Saeed M, Hanna I, Robotis D, Styperek R, Polosajian L, Khan A, et al. Programming implantable cardioverter-defibrillators in patients with primary prevention indication to prolong time to first shock: Results from the PROVIDE study. Journal of Cardiovascular Electrophysiology. 2014;**25**(1):52-59

[32] Kusumoto FM, Calkins H, BoehmerJ, et al. Heart rhythm society; American college of cardiology; American Heart Association. HRS/ACC/AHA expert consensus statement on the use of implantable cardioverter-defibrillator therapy in patients who are not included or not well represented in clinical trials. Journal of the American College of Cardiology. 2014;**64**(11):1143-1177

Section 3

Advances in Endocardial Signal Processing

Chapter 8

Complexity of Atrial Fibrillation Electrograms Through Nonlinear Signal Analysis: In Silico Approach

Catalina Tobón, Andrés Orozco-Duque,
Juan P. Ugarte, Miguel Becerra and Javier Saiz

Additional information is available at the end of the chapter

http://dx.doi.org/10.5772/intechopen.69475

Abstract

Identification of atrial fibrillation (AF) mechanisms could improve the rate of ablation success. However, the incomplete understanding of those mechanisms makes difficult the decision of targeting sites for ablation. This work is focused on the importance of EGM analysis for detecting and modulating rotors to guide ablation procedures and improve its outcomes. Virtual atrial models are used to show how nonlinear measures can be used to generate electroanatomical maps to detect critical sites in AF. A description of the atrial cell mathematical models, and the procedure of coupling them within two-dimensional and three-dimensional virtual atrial models in order to simulate arrhythmogenic mechanisms, is given. Mathematical modeling of unipolar and bipolar electrogramas (EGM) is introduced. It follows a discussion of EGM signal processing. Nonlinear descriptors, such as approximate entropy and multifractal analysis, are used to study the dynamical behavior of EGM signals, which are not well described by a linear law. Our results evince that nonlinear analysis of EGM can provide information about the dynamics of rotors and other mechanisms of AF. Furthermore, these fibrillatory patterns can be simulated using virtual models. The combination of features using machine learning tools can be used for identifying arrhythmogenic sources of AF.

Keywords: atrial fibrillation, arrhythmogenic sources, electrogram model, computer simulation, nonlinear features, electroanatomical mapping

1. Introduction

The most common sustained cardiac arrhythmias in humans are associated with the atria. Atrial arrhythmias, mainly atrial fibrillation (AF), frequently provoke incapacitating symptoms and severe complications such as stroke and heart failure [1]. Overall, 20–25% of all strokes are caused by AF [2]. The presence of AF is related to a significant increase in morbidity and mortality [3]. Electrocardiogram-based surveys suggest that 1% of the total population is affected by AF [4].

There are a large number of clinical conditions that are associated with an increased incidence of AF. This contributes to a progressive process of atrial remodeling characterized by a set of changes in atrial properties that contributes in sustaining of the arrhythmia. These changes include alterations in the electrical cellular activity, calcium handling and in the atrial structure such as cellular hypertrophy and fibrosis. They have been described in some animal models [5–8] and in humans [9–11]. These alterations may favor the occurrence of triggers that initiate the AF and the formation of a substrate that promotes its perpetuation. Changes in electrical activity cause a significant shortening of the action potential duration (APD) and a decrease in refractoriness [8–10], which may support the initiation and maintenance of multiple re-entrant waves, as suggested by experimental studies [5, 9].

It is well known that AF can be caused by different mechanisms, including single-circuit re-entry, multiple-circuit re-entry, rapid local ectopic activity and rotors [12–15]. It is very important to know the mechanisms underlying AF, since these have implications in the treatment of the disease. An important percentage of patients suffers of paroxysmal AF, which is initiated by focal triggers that are localized at preferential sites, mainly in the pulmonary veins (PV) [13]. Electrical isolation of pulmonary veins can prevent recurrence of AF in 70–80% of these lone AF patients. The rationale for this is the crucial observation, reported in [13], that AF was mostly triggered by ectopic beats arising from the muscle sleeves of the pulmonary veins. They demonstrated that atrial rapid paces or ectopic activity originated in the proximities or in the interior of the pulmonary veins could act like triggers, and, in some cases, they would be responsible for the maintenance of paroxysmal AF episodes [16, 17]. A unifying theory suggests that rapid focal activity is responsible for generating atrial, which is necessary to maintain a substrate for the generation of multiple re-entrant waves [18, 19]. While paroxysmal AF is maintained predominantly by ectopic focal activity or local re-entrant circuits located in one or more pulmonary veins, as the arrhythmia evolves into more persistent forms promoted by atrial remodeling, the mechanisms that maintain AF move toward the atria and are increasingly based on re-entry substrates [11, 20–22]. Based on clinical [23–25] and experimental [14, 26] results, certain types of AF can be attributed to a stable high-frequency rotor or a small number of rotor waves in left atrium, which maintain the arrhythmia, whose periodic activation can be converted into a chaotic pattern when the wavefronts propagate across the atrial wall. This phenomenon, known as the *mother rotor hypothesis*, is the most recently proposed mechanism of AF [27], which suggests that AF is triggered by a series of ectopic beats, whose wave fronts give rise to a rotor. The rotor is a stable re-entry around a functionally unexcitable core [15] that works as a maintenance mechanism with some spatial temporal stability, activating the local tissue at high frequency, generating wave fronts that fragment and propagate as multiple daughter wavelets. Stable rotors are at diverse locations, mostly in the left atrium, including sites outside the pulmonary veins, as well as the posterior, inferior, and roof regions. Several studies have observed rotors in in vitro and animal models [14, 28, 29], and its presence in humans has been reported [27, 30, 31].

All localized sources of AF as re-entry circuits, ectopic foci, or rotors, cause fibrillatory conduction remote from the source, which is difficult to distinguish from propagation that maintains the AF by multiple wavelets, and any of these phenomena may generate rotors registered by intracardiac recordings [32, 24]. Studies carried out by [33, 34] have shown evidence that human AF can be sustained by localized rotors; however, the existence of stable rotors maintaining AF remains a focus of discussion. Hence, the importance of the implementation of virtual models and computational tools in the studies of AF sources and its relation with the signals recorded from surface. In the same way, the rotors have been shown in computer models of AF [35–38].

Ablation has emerged as an important treatment strategy for AF [39]. Pulmonary veins isolation reaches single procedure success rates of 60–80% for paroxysmal AF treatment [40]. However, for the chronic case, this strategy does not achieve satisfactory outcomes [41]; consequently, complex ablation lines are added to the procedure [45]. Catheter ablation guided by electroanatomic mapping has revolutionized the treatment of permanent AF. Identification of AF mechanisms could improve the rate of ablation success. However, the incomplete understanding of those mechanisms makes difficult the decision of targeting sites for ablation. To overcome this limitation, two-dimensional and realistic three-dimensional human atria computer models have been developed to investigate the relationship between the characteristics of EGM and the propagation pattern associated with them [42–45].

It is thought that the different mechanisms lead to changes in the characteristics of spatiotemporal organization of AF [44, 45]. EGM-guided ablation procedures have been proposed as an alternative strategy, which involves mapping and ablating focal sources or complex fractionated atrial electrograms (CFAE) [46]. Recent studies have shown that a large number of sites representing AF substrates are characterized by a high degree of disorganization in EGM signals [29], and therefore, signal processing methods are being designed in order to quantify their degree of fractionation [47, 48]. The relationship between the rotor tip and CFAE has been published in recent studies [36, 45, 47, 49, 50]; however, automatic rotor mapping methods have not been fully developed.

Different mapping techniques are being used to identify target sites for ablation, and some of them are activation waves, voltage, dominant frequency [23, 51–55] and CFAE maps [39, 46, 56]. Nevertheless, there are several limitations with these techniques, and one of the most important is that they depend considerably on the electrophysiologist expertise [57].

The term CFAE was introduced by Nademanee [46] as a pathophysiological concept; however, its definition is unclear and broad and includes inherent subjectivity [58]. CFAE are formally defined as follows: (1) atrial EGM that have fractionated electrograms composed of two deflections or more, and/or perturbation of the baseline with continuous deflection of a prolonged activation complex over a 10 s recording period; (2) atrial EGM with a very short cycle length (<120 ms) over a 10 s recording period. CFAE definition does not distinguish between different morphologies; consequently, fractionated EGM according with CFAE definition are not necessarily related to arrhythmogenic substrates. Moreover, several studies have shown conflicting results with Nademanee [56, 59]. This may lead the electrophysiologist to confuse the fractionated EGM that are functional in nature [60] with fractionated EGM corresponding to arrhythmogenic sources, leading to incorrect target sites for ablation. This also makes clinical results difficult to compare. Inconsistent results have been found in different studies using the CFAE concept. Although the concept of CFAE has made a great contribution to the study of AF, it may fail to describe the wide range of fractionation that occurs in the EGM signals in specific cases. Thus, the electrogram-guided approach by mapping and targeting areas of CFAE is a technique that is still debated [61], and further studies are needed to strengthen the treatment techniques.

To date, indexes computation from EGM is carried out mostly based on the detection of local activation waves and time intervals. However, the concept of EGM fractionation, such as CFAE, defined using time criteria, is not enough to describe the complexity of EGM during AF. Morphological irregularity and temporal variability of the signal must be included. To overcome the limitations of CFAE definition, designation of different degree of fractionation has been proposed based on the perturbation of baseline and the presence of continuous deflection [36]. Some studies have presented evidence linking the vortex of the rotor with a high degree of fractionation in the EGM [36, 47]. However, the patterns of EGM signals associated with the rotors are still unknown, and the development of tools for characterizing fractionated EGM signals is still a current topic. In addition, there is not a standard for description of fractionation degrees, and there are different descriptions in the literature. In order to quantify the behavior of different morphologies of EGM signals and the fractionation degrees, recent studies have helped to understand the concept of EGM fractionation as a nonlinear phenomenon [47, 48, 62]. Mathematical descriptors of the nonlinear dynamical behavior have been used to study cardiac signals and are based on the description of the state of the system and its evolution. If a linear law does not describe the evolution of the system, the dynamics is nonlinear. Thus, indexes and features calculated using nonlinear dynamics theory become an alternative for enhancing assessment of EGM complexity.

2. Simulated atrial fibrillation dynamics

The mathematical modeling of atrial electrophysiology has become a useful method for studying the underlying mechanisms responsible for AF. Different models of human atrial electrophysiology have been published with various formulations of ionic currents and calcium handling, therefore, with different electrophysiological properties [63–67]. In our studies, the transmembrane potential was based on the Courtemanche-Ramirez-Nattel and Kneller [63, 68] model of human atrial cell kinetics in the presence of 0.005 μM of acetylcholine (ACh). Based on the experimental data [9, 10, 69], the cell model was modified in order to reproduce electrophysiological conditions of permanent AF: the maximum conductance of delayed rectifier potassium current (I_{Kur}) and transient potassium current (I_{to}) was decreased by 50%, the maximum conductance of potassium time independent current (I_{K1}) was increased by 100%, and the maximum conductance of L-type calcium current (I_{CaL}) was decreased by 70% (see **Table 1**). Thus, the action potential duration at 90% of the repolarization (APD90) was reduced by 70% (**Figure 1A**), which is in accordance with experimental studies developed by Workman et al. [9] and Bosch et al. [10] in isolated myocytes from patients with permanent AF, using the whole cell patch clamp technique.

The development of multi-dimensional models has allowed representing fibers, pieces of tissue and atrial cavities. These models have served to approach, among other aspects, the biophysics of the action potential propagation under physiological and pathological conditions.

Different studies have developed and implemented two-dimensional (2D) models of atrial tissue to study the action potential propagation dynamics under physiological and pathological conditions [36, 37, 68, 70].

We have developed a two-dimensional model of human atrial tissue. The tissue surface was discretized into a 150 × 150 hexahedral mesh (22,500 elements and 45,602 nodes). Spatial resolution was 0.4 mm. The electrical propagation of the atrial action potential was modeled using the monodomain reaction–diffusion equation:

$$\frac{1}{S_v}\nabla\cdot\left(D\nabla V_m\right) = C_m\frac{\partial V_m}{\partial t} + I_{ion} - I_{stim} \tag{1}$$

where S_v corresponds to the surface-to-volume ratio, D is the conductivity tensor, C_m is the specific membrane capacitance (50 pF), I_{ion} is the total ionic current that crosses the membrane cells, V_m is the membrane potential, and I_{stim} is the stimulus current. The electrophysiological model was integrated into the two-dimensional virtual model. The equation was solved using the EMOS software, which is a parallel code that implements the finite element method and operator splitting [42, 71] for solving the monodomain model of electrical propagation and allows to calculate EGM as postprocess. The time step was fixed to 0.001 ms.

The tissue was considered isotropic. A conductivity of 0.3 S/cm was assigned to obtain a realistic conduction velocity of 60 cm/s.

Rotor was generated by S1–S2 cross-field stimulation protocol. Stimuli pulses were rectangular with 2 ms of duration and 6 mA of amplitude. The S1 was a train of five plane stimuli applied at the left boundary of the model at a basic cycle length of 1000 ms. The S2 stimulus was rectangular (3 × 2 cm) and was applied 40 ms after the last S1 in the inferior left corner of the model (**Figure 1B**).

A 4s stable clockwise spiral wave (rotor) was observed in the two-dimensional model after applying the protocol (**Figure 1C**). The APD shortening due to the atrial remodeling allowed the rotor stability over time. Wijffels et al. [8] in goats demonstrated that maintenance of AF by pacing in the normal goat heart resulted in the development of sustained AF within 1–3 weeks. This observation of tachycardia-induced electrical remodeling creating a background for persistent AF led to the concept that "Atrial Fibrillation Begets Atrial Fibrillation." The longer duration and stability of the AF episodes was explained by a shortening of the wavelength of the atrial impulse. The simulated rotor pattern agrees with the "rotor hypothesis" proposed by Jalife [15]. The contour map was implemented to show the core of the rotor (circular point in **Figure 1D**).

Virtual models of cardiac structures are needed in the study of atrial arrhythmias that are critically dependent on the spatial organization of cardiac structures and fibers. Some atrial

Conductance	Permanent AF
gI_{KL}	Increased by 100%
gI_{KACh}	–
gI_{Kuv}	Decreased by 50%
gI_{to}	Decreased by 50%
gI_{CaL}	Decreased by 70%

Table 1. Conductance (g) changes of currents for permanent AF.

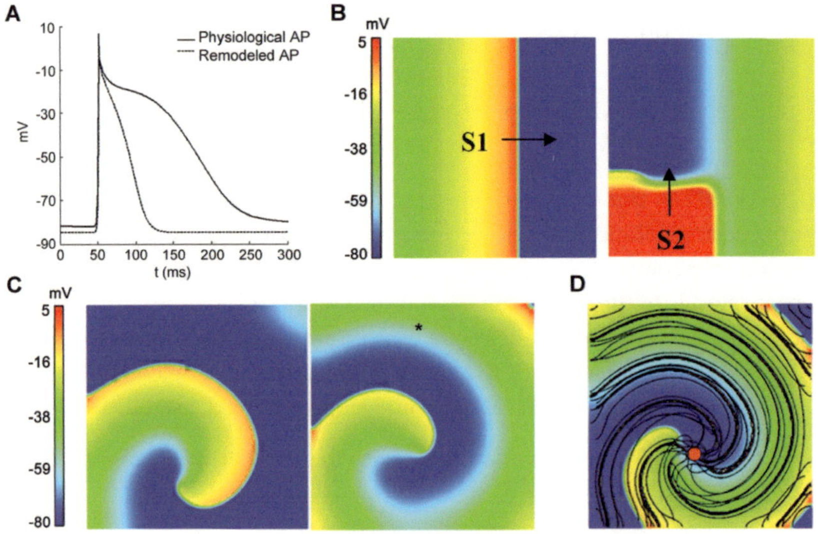

Figure 1. (A) Action potential under physiological and permanent AF conditions. (B) S1–S2 cross-field protocol. The plane S1 and rectangular S2 stimulus are shown. (C) Stable rotor under permanent AF conditions. (D) Contour map, the circular point indicates the rotor tip location.

arrhythmias, such as AF, need complete structures to perpetuate them. The validity and enormous potential of multi-scale heart models in improving diagnosis, prevention and therapy of cardiac pathologies are supported by different scientific results. These virtual models have opened new horizons in the study of the complex mechanisms underlying atrial arrhythmias and their treatment, either pharmacological or surgical. The earliest complex atrial models incorporated parts of the anatomical architecture of the atria [72, 73]. During the last few years, a significant number of new models of the animal and human atrial anatomy have been published [44, 74–88]. Some of these models included the atrial fiber architecture observed in histological sections. Studies developed by Seemann et al. [75] and Aslanidi et al. [79] included only the main bundles fiber orientation in their human atrial model. An image-based anatomical model of the sheep atrial has been published [80] including realistic fiber orientation. The model reproduces the whole atria with highly detailed myofiber architecture.

The three-dimensional models also allow relating the arrhythmic behaviors as focal activity, rotors and multiple wavelet reentries, with their manifestation in the electrograms [44, 81].

A realistic three-dimensional model of human atria including the main anatomical structures (**Figure 2A**), electrophysiological heterogeneity, anisotropy (conduction velocity in the direction of myocardial fibers is usually several times larger than that vertical to them), and fiber orientation (**Figure 2B**) was developed in an earlier work [42]. It includes 52,906 hexahedral elements (polyhedrons with six faces, eight corners or nodes, topologically equivalent to cubes). The mathematical atrial cell model coupled within three-dimensional (3D) virtual atria model was used to simulate AF dynamics. AF episodes were generated by the S1–S2 stimulation protocol as follows [36]: a train of five stimuli with a basic cycle length of 1000 ms was applied in the sinus node area for a period of 5 s to simulate the atrial sinus rhythm (S1). Based on the study developed by Haissaguerre et al. [13], a burst pacing of 6 ectopic beats to high frequency (S2) at cycle length (CL) of 130 ms was delivered into the right superior pulmonary vein after the last S1.

During AF activity initiated by the ectopic activity, it was observed the generation of two rotors of stable activity during 5 s of simulation. One was located in the posterior wall of the left atrium, near the left pulmonary vein (#2 in **Figure 2D**), and the other was located in the superior vena cava (#1 in **Figure 2D**). The rotors were generated spontaneously, which is in agreement with the rotor hypothesis [27]. Additionally, a block line located over the inferior right pulmonary vein has been observed (#3 in **Figure 2D**).

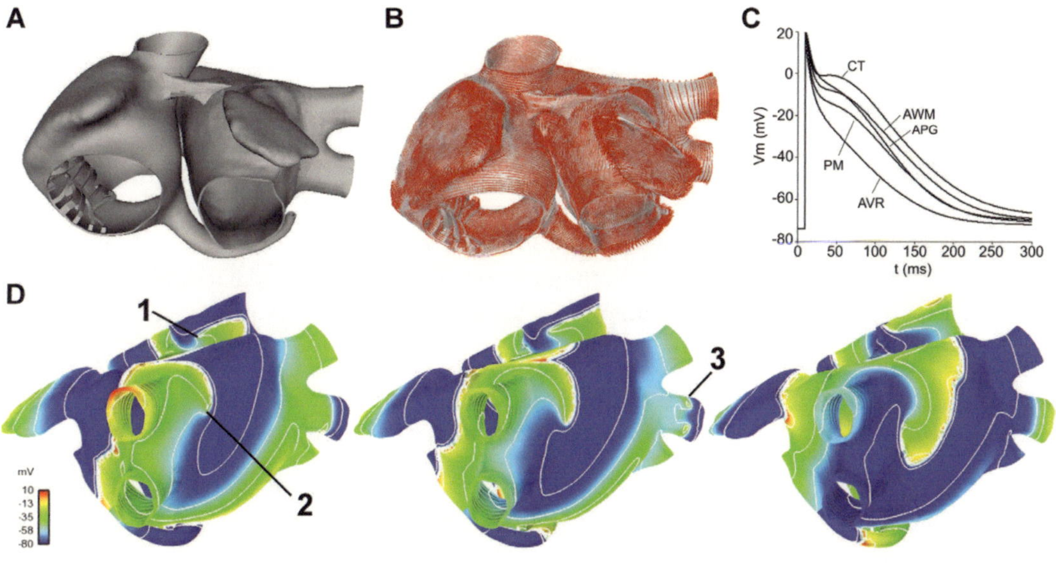

Figure 2. (A) Frontal view of the three-dimensional model of human atria. (B) Fiber orientation. (C) AP for different atrial areas (CT: crista terminalis, PM: pectinate muscles, APG: appendages, AVR: atrioventricular rings, and AWM: atrial working myocardium) under physiological conditions. (D) Activation isochronal maps. Stable rotors located in the posterior wall of the left atrium (#2) and A in the superior vena cava (#1) are showed. A block line can be seen at the right inferior pulmonary vein (#3).

3. Simulated atrial electrograms

Several studies [21, 60, 82–84] have investigated the effects of factors such as slow conduction, anisotropy, conduction blocks, re-entries, and wave collisions, on the morphology of unipolar and bipolar EGM. However, it is still not entirely clear to what extent these factors contribute to temporal and spatial variations in EGM morphology as observed during AF.

Calculating atrial EGM from the virtual models allows the study of EGM morphology and their relationship with arrhythmogenic sources.

Unipolar EGM are modeled as the register of the extracellular potential measured by a positive polarity electrode whose reference (zero potential) is located at infinity. The distance from the electrode to the surface quantifies the influence area of the electrode, so the closer it is to the tissue, the greater the field uptake. The extracellular potential (Φ_e) was computed using the large volume conductor approximation [85, 86]:

$$\phi_e(r) = -K\iiint \nabla' V_m(r') \cdot \nabla'\left[\frac{1}{r'-r}\right]dv \tag{2}$$

where K is a constant that includes the ratio of intracellular and extracellular conductivities ($\sigma_i/4\pi\,\sigma_e$), $\nabla' V_m$ is the spatial gradient of transmembrane potential V_m, r is the distance from the source point (x, y, z) to the measuring point (x', y', z') and dv is the differential volume.

Zlochiver et al. [45] investigated the regularity of EGM in the presence of stable rotors, in a two-dimensional atrial model. Jacquemet et al. [87] in a computer model representing a monolayer of atrial cells concluded that microscale obstacles cause significant changes to EGM waveforms. Using two-dimensional computer models and cell cultures, Navoret et al. [88] detected CFAE using the criteria of cycle length, number of deflections, and amplitude. They established a relationship between the detected CFAE and the presence of rotors and shock waves, but they failed to differentiate them. Ashihara et al. [89], using a two-dimensional myocardial sheet of size 4.5 × 4.5 cm, studied the role of fibroblasts in CFAE during AF. Yun et al. [90] reported that CFAE in a homogeneous two-dimensional AF model were weakly correlated with wave break, phase singularity, and local dominant frequency.

We simulated that in the two-dimensional atrial model, a total of 22,500 virtual electrodes (150 × 150, one for each element of the model), spaced by 0.4 mm at a distance of 0.2 mm above the atrial surface, unipolar EGM were calculated with temporal resolution of 1 ms.

The 98.9% of EGM, located away from the rotor tip, present simple morphology (**Figure 3A**). The remaining 1.1% of EGM, located at the rotor tip, exhibits potentials composed by two or more deflections (**Figure 3B**).

The mechanism by which fractionation of unipolar EGM occurs in our simulations can be explained as follows: the rotor is a singularity point or phase singularity, when the rotor is stable it pivots around a circular trajectory forming the core of the spiral wave, afterwards the pivot point is affected by the wavefronts from the rotor tip. When the wavefront passes near to the pivot point in each rotation cycle, several electrotonic potentials (nonpropagated local potential) are observed; consequently, irregularity and fractionation arise [36]. Our results are consistent with other studies, in which unipolar EGM symmetry was affected by the wavefront curvature (convex, concave or amorphous) [44] and fractionated unipolar EGM were observed at pivot points (functionally unexcitable core around which the rotor turns) [82]. Umapathy et al. [50] reported that CFAE were located in the region of a rotor tip and sites where wave breaks, using a murine HL-1 atrial monolayer model.

Most of the in silico studies using three-dimensional atrial models have characterized the simulated arrhythmias by observing the re-entrant patterns. Few authors [44] have also calculated EGM in a circular region on the free wall of the right atrium, using the 16 unipolar virtual electrodes on a simplified three-dimensional model of human atria. They suggested that analysis of the amplitude and symmetry of unipolar atrial electrograms can provide information about the electrophysiological substrate maintaining AF. Hwang et al. [81] calculated bipolar EGM in a personalized three-dimensional left atrial model in order to applied virtual ablation at CFAE points.

We calculated 42,835 EGM in the whole atrial surface of the three-dimensional atrial model, over a 4-s window and recorded at 1 kHz. Bipolar EGM were calculated by subtracting two 1 mm-spaced adjacent unipolar EGM.

Fractionated atrial EGM were shown to be located in rotor tip areas, when the tip of the rotor turned on this point, displaying low voltage and irregular morphology with potentials composed by two or more deflections (**Figure 4A** and **B**). The wavefront of the rotor surrounds the pivot point, without depolarizing it completely, which results in multiple low amplitude deflections in the EGM.

The EGM corresponding to the block line present fractionation; however, the activation patterns are visible, and their amplitudes are similar to nonfractionated EGM (**Figure 4C**). The EGM from sites with a plain wavefront are regular with potentials composed by one deflection (**Figure 4D**).

We identified the area in the posterior wall of the left atrium where the rotor spins (shaded circle in **Figure 5A**). EGM signals obtained from this area were used. From the selected region of the model, a conversion was made from the three-dimensional coordinate system to the two-dimensional coordinate system (x, z), taking advantage of the very low dispersion in y. EGM were converted to bipolar EGM, and this task was accomplished by creating a virtual mesh with 1 mm spacing, and performing a match with the two-dimensional model surface. In this way, the difference between two adjacent signals in the mesh was calculated, obtaining a bipolar signal. In the same way, the results show that the rotor vortex area is associated with

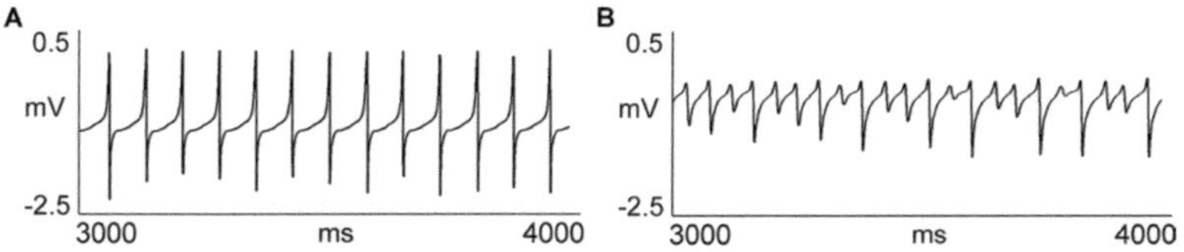

Figure 3. (A) Regular EGM calculated in '*' from **Figure 1C**. (B) Fractionated EGM calculated in the rotor tip.

signals presenting high degree of fractionation (**Figure 5B**). For the contrary, the EGM from sites with a plain wavefront are regular with potentials composed by one deflection, similarly to the unipolar EGM morphology (**Figure 5C**).

4. Estimation of nonlinear features for electroanatomical mapping

EGM-guided ablation has been proposed as a strategy to find critical sites of AF as target sites for ablation. Multiple clinical trials have shown that ablation of fractionated electrograms adds no benefit to conventional AF ablation with pulmonary vein isolation [91, 92]. This is likely because sites of electrogram fractionation, according with CFAE definition, not always correlate with sites of arrhythmic drivers and can also represent sites of wavefront collision or slow conduction, among others. Although CFAE may be relevant to detect areas that maintain AF, further characteristics apart from fractionation should be important to identify the atrial sites that maintain AF.

To overcome the limitation of CFAE, nonlinear analysis of EGM signals has been proposed by several authors to analyze the signals using further characteristics apart from time intervals or number of deflection [93, 94]. Nonlinear features are studied using the raw EGM signals, and it is not necessary to detect local activation waves. This is an important property, because in fragmented signals detection of activation waves is not always feasible. Nonlinear features

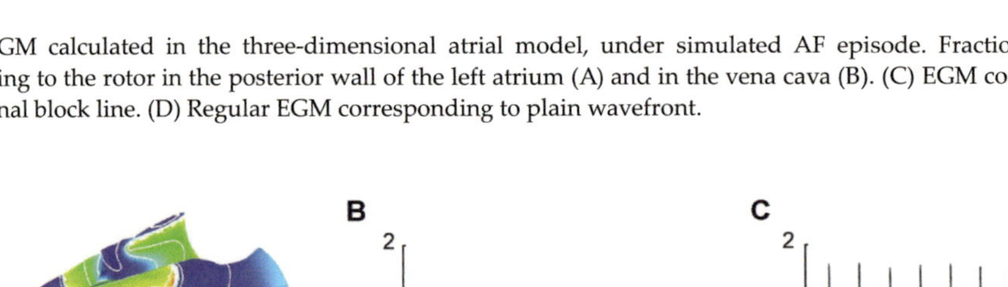

Figure 4. EGM calculated in the three-dimensional atrial model, under simulated AF episode. Fractionated EGM corresponding to the rotor in the posterior wall of the left atrium (A) and in the vena cava (B). (C) EGM corresponding to a functional block line. (D) Regular EGM corresponding to plain wavefront.

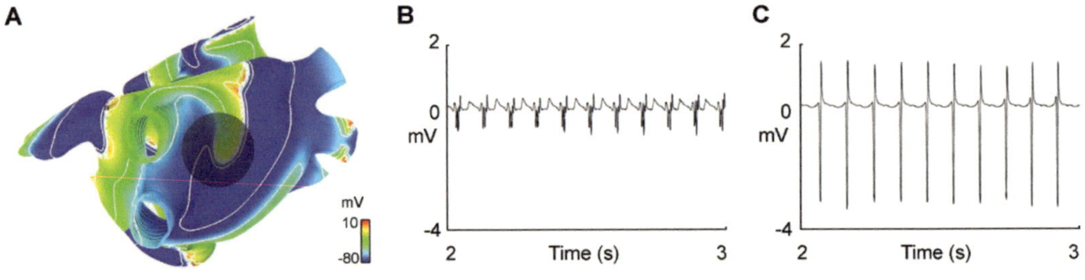

Figure 5. (A) The area in the posterior wall in the model to obtain bipolar EGM. Samples of two bipolar EGM are shown, a fractionated signal from the rotor tip (B) and a regular activation pattern from nonrotor area (C).

as entropy estimation and fractal analysis are compute over each single EGM, and its value is related to the complexity of the signal.

Nonlinear mathematical tools can be used to quantify the irregularity of a signal. During the last years, measures have been developed to estimate the complexity of biomedical signals. Main goal of these advancements is to provide new theories about the dynamics of biological systems. Such is the case of Kolmogorov-Sinai entropy, Lempel-Ziv complexity, and correlation dimension, among others [95]. However, most of the complexity indexes require long time series to obtain reliable and convergent measures. Pincus [96] proposed the statistic approximate entropy (*ApEn*), which solves the issue of short time series, and it is aimed to measure the complexity degree and the presence of similarity patterns. Further developments have followed the *ApEn*, taking this as a starting point, such as the sample entropy [97], the fuzzy entropy [98] or hierarchical entropy [99]. Some authors have reported the use of nonlinear features to evaluate their suitable for locating critical sites in AF. For instances, Ganesas et al. [47] reported that sites near to the rotor tip present high values of Shannon Entropy (*ShEn*) in EGM signals recorded from cell cultures and simulated episodes of fibrillatory conduction in two-dimensional models of atrial tissue.

4.1. Approximate and Shannon entropy definitions

In general words, entropy has been conceived as a measure of the degree of disorganization or irregularity of a process. The most organized the process is, the lower the entropy related to it.

The statistic $ApEn(m, r, N)$ depends on the length N of the time series $x(n)$ (where n is), the positive integer m (where $m \le N$) and the positive real number r. Defining:

$$\Phi^m(r) = \frac{\sum_{i=1}^{N-m+1} \log[\, C_i^m(r)\,]}{N-(m-1)} \tag{3}$$

we have that $ApEn(m, r, N) = \Phi^m(r) - \Phi^{m+1}(r)$.

The variable $C_i^m(r)$ counts the number of segments of length m that are within the boundaries defined by r. Thus, *ApEn(m, r, N)* measures the logarithmic frequency of the tool measures the logarithmic frequency that those segments of length m that are close remain close after increasing the length of the segments by one. In such a way, the statistic *ApEn* provides a measure of irregularity of the signal, implying strong regularity when *ApEn* value is small, and irregularity when *ApEn* value is large [96].

In previous work, we have reported the use of *ApEn* to evaluate the location of rotors and block lines in a three-dimensional model of human atrial [100]; and the use of multifractal analysis as a tool to discriminate between four levels of fractionation according with a modified Well's approach [101]. In this work, we tested several nonlinear features using EGM signals recorded from a two-dimensional model of atrial tissue and a three-dimensional model of human atrial. Additional, we test the used of combination of nonlinear features using clustering method to study the distribution of different EGM patterns over the atrial surface.

Another index that estimates the entropy value from an N-point signal $x(n)$ is Shannon entropy (*ShE*) defined as:

$$ShEn = -\sum_{i=1}^{N} p_i \log_2(p_i)$$

where p_i is the probability of assuming the corresponding *x(i)* value. Both, *ApEn* and *ShEn*, consider that a high value of repeated patterns implies order. Thus, they make their respective estimations of a signal irregularity by counting repetitive patterns, where the *ApEn* has a more elaborate method of defining and counting these patterns.

4.2. Nonlinear features to complexity estimation for building maps: two-dimensional model case

Nonlinear features such as *ShEn* and *ApEn* have been used and tested for locating stables rotors in simulated episodes of fibrillatory conduction. We have tested *ShEn* maps and *ApEn* maps using the EGM signals from the two-dimensional model. Results of this approach are shown in **Figure 6A** and **E**. These maps are constructed with high resolution using all the signals available in the model: 22,500 with spatial resolution of 0.4 mm. However, in the real case, the resolution of the electrodes can be lower, so in Ref. [102] was carried out a study about the EGM maps analysis reducing their resolution. **Figure 6** shows the maps of two-dimensional model of AF reconstructed from the entire model with a 75% of reduction of the electrodes number (resolution: 37 × 38) and characterized using the features *ShEn* and *ApEn* of the EGM signals, respectively. A reconstruction of the entire model was developed using the interpolation techniques: Inverse distance weighted -IDW [103] (**Figure 6B** and **F**), IDW with Mean Filter–MF [104] (**Figure 6C** and **G**), and backpropagation artificial neural network—BPANN (**Figure 6D** and **H**). The best result is obtained with BPANN algorithm. Backpropagation artificial neural network (BPANN) is a type of artificial neural network that assumes the function of a common and complex nervous system, and BPANN is widely used in machine learning for clinical research [105, 106]. BPANN is trained using Levenberg-Marquardt backpropagation algorithm [107]. This technique was applied for predicting the

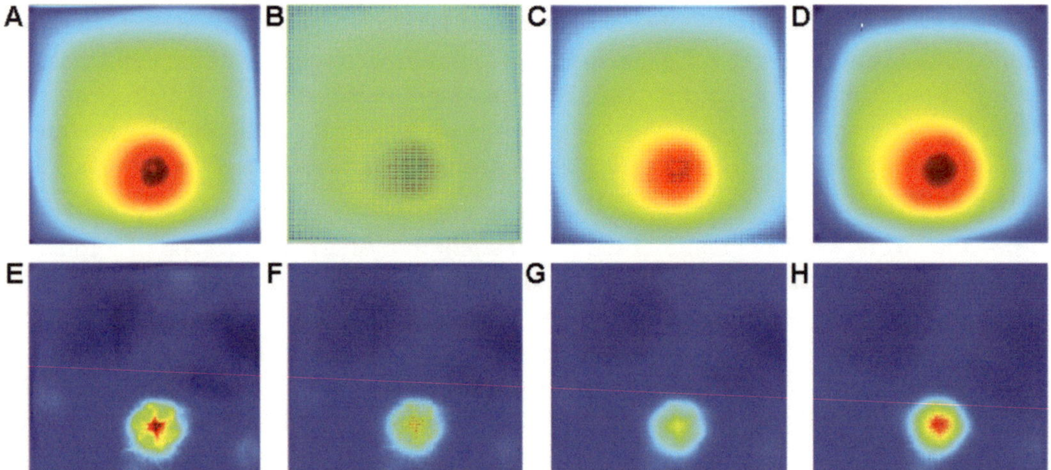

Figure 6. (A) Two-dimensional ShEn map. ShEn map reconstructed 75% using IDW-MF (B) and BPANN (C). (D) Log entropy map. (E) Two-dimensional ApEn map. ApEn map reconstructed 75% using IDW-MF (F) and BPANN (G). (H) Log entropy map.

values of unknown points in order to increase the resolution of the two-dimensional Map. BPANN has a structure (layers and neurons—[2 5 4 3 2 1]), which was defined applying a heuristic adjustment based on the minimum error for the mean map. The performance was assessed using the root mean squared error (RMSE).

5. Approximate entropy for rotor detection: three-dimensional model case

Motivated by the features of the *ApEn*, as a signal analyzing tool, and its important presence in several studies of complex biological systems [108–113]; our group has performed a study that relates AF mechanisms, such as rotors, with high degree of irregularity of EGM by means of the *ApEn*. In the following sections, *ApEn* theoretical definition and its interpretation are presented. Moreover, *ApEn* electroanatomical maps obtained from the virtual models are presented, as well as the feasibility of characterize fibrillatory mechanisms in space and time. It follows a detailed analysis of our results and their implications.

5.1. Approximate entropy for locating critical sites in AF

As stated earlier, our group has performed numerical experiments to assess the regularity of atrial EGM signals by means of the *ApEn*. Our research is based on three hypotheses: (1) Fractionation of EGM increases the *ApEn* values. (2) High *ApEn* values can be related to the tip of a rotor. (3) Information about spatial and temporal dynamics of a rotor could be obtained using moving window *ApEn*.

In order to calculate the *ApEn* values from the virtual unipolar EGM, we define the parameters $m = 2$ and $r = 0.1$ according to the interval of values suggested by Pincus [96], and $N = 1000$. **Figure 1** shows three EGM of 1000 points each, corresponding to minimum, intermediate and maximum *ApEn* values. The *ApEn* corresponds with the morphological complexity of the EGM: High values of *ApEn* mean irregularity or fragmentation of the EGM, and vice versa. In **Figure 7**, the EGM of the bottom present fragmentation of activation waves and baseline irregularity. Intermediate values of *ApEn* represent transitions between nonfragmented and fragmented EGM, in which differences between the patterns of activation waves can be seen, as can be seen in the EGM of the middle.

Figure 8 (middle) shows the electroanatomical map of *ApEn(2, 0.1, 1000)* for the first second of the episode. The areas of R1 and R2, right inferior pulmonary vein and coronary sinus, have high *ApEn* values (red). The *ApEn* values (green) increase in the appendix, in pulmonary veins, and on the posterior and inferior wall of the left atrium. Rotors are established at the R1 and R2 zones. The high *ApEn* regions in **Figure 8** are not specifically related to rotor activity. Some authors suggest that the standard *ApEn* parameters are not suitable for signals of fast dynamics, and that to solve these cases, the *r* and *m* parameters must be chosen from a larger set than the one proposed by Pincus [108, 114]. Following this idea, we designed an optimization process for the *ApEn* parameters obtaining the configuration *ApEn(3, 0.38, 1000)*. **Figure 8** (right) shows the corresponding *ApEn* in which the rotors R1 and R2 are highlighted by high *ApEn* values. Moreover, intermediate values of *ApEn* (green) are related to perturbations in conduction such as blockades, at the right inferior pulmonary vein, and shockwaves, at the zone below the coronary sinus. For additional details of this procedure and the results please refer to Ref. [115].

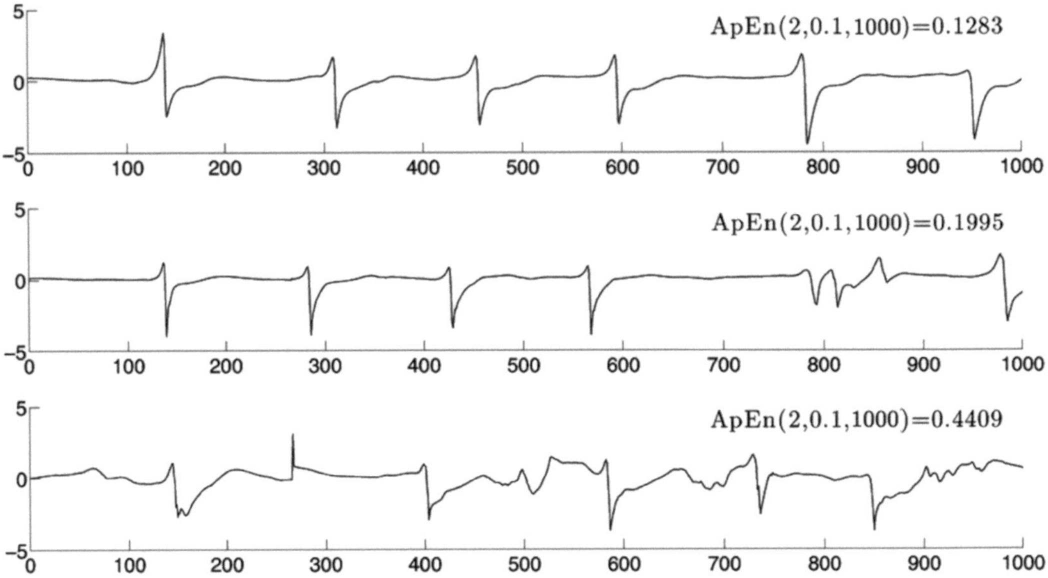

Figure 7. Three degrees of EGM irregularity and the corresponding ApEn value.

The fibrillatory activity presented in **Figure 8** includes stable rotors that were characterized by the *ApEn* maps. We move now to the case in which the tip of the rotor meanders. To gain in temporal resolution, the parameter *N* was reduced to 500 points, and a nonoverlapping moving window was applied to each EGM of the model to obtain a time-dependent *ApEn* value (**Figure 9**). We applied Pincus parameters *ApEn(2,0.1,500)* and optimized parameters *ApEn(2,0.3,500)*. The analysis is performed over window of observation located at the left atrial posterior wall, in which a meandering rotor is generated. **Figure 10** shows three consecutive frames of the episode (firs two columns) and the *ApEn* electroanatomical maps for Pincus (third column) and optimized (fourth column) parameters. For both parameter configuration, the high *ApEn* region changes as the tip of the rotor meanders through the observation window. The bottom row shows no rotor within the window that induces a reduction of *ApEn* for optimized parameters, while for Pincus parameters, high *ApEn* values remain.

Under the assumptions of our computational model, we provide evidence that the hypotheses stated above: we are able to quantify fragmentation of EGM using the *ApEn* as a measure of regularity and to relate it with the tip of a stable and meandering rotors. Moreover, through an optimized version of *ApEn* parameters setup, other conduction anomalies can be identified. There are several works, with similar approach but with different tools of measurement of irregularity [54, 26, 88, 116, 50]. The tools used for the fragmentation analysis are mostly based on the calculation of the length of the cycle and the amplitude of the EGM, in correspondence with the definition of Nademanee [46]. Although the concept of CFAE established by Nademanee has been an important contribution to the study of AF, it may not describe the wide range of EGM fragmentations that occur in different cases. Therefore, we propose to extend the concept of fragmentation as a nonstatic and nonlinear phenomenon. The *ApEn* has already been applied in other studies for EGM analysis in AF [117], and in ventricular fibrillation [118]

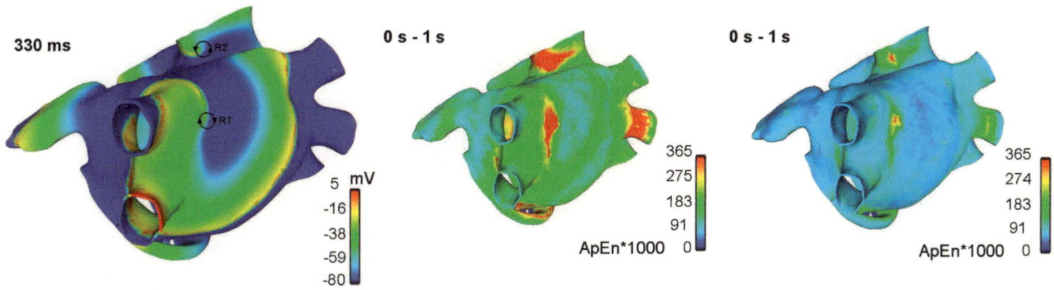

Figure 8. ApEn electroanatomical maps for AF episode. The notations R1 and R2 correspond to the tip of rotors at the left atrial posterior wall and superior cava vein.

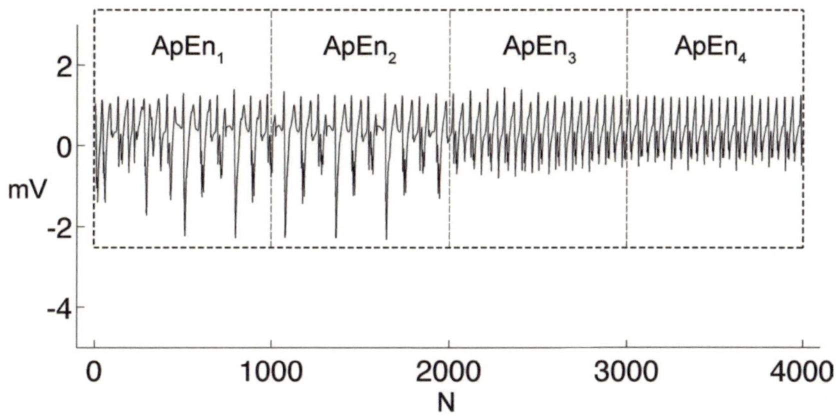

Figure 9. Nonoverlapping moving window procedure to obtain ApEn values varying in time.

obtaining a single *ApEn* value for each EGM signal. We applied the Dynamic *ApEn* using a mobile window of 500 and 1000 points. An EGM of 4 s can provide up to 8 *ApEn* values, aimed to gain temporal resolution, and information about the behavior of EGM fragmentation.

The fragmented EGM were characterized by means of the *ApEn*, using the standard parameters suggested by Pincus and the parameters chosen from the proposed optimization method [115]. Both proposals reveal the relationship between CFAE and high values of *ApEn*, which is supported by Novak et al. [94]. Furthermore, EGM fragments with high *ApEn* values have been shown to be related to arrhythmogenic substrates, such as the rotor tip, blocking lines and the case of the coronary sinus area influenced by abrupt fiber direction, wave collision and passage from a narrow conducting zone to a wide but perpendicular zone. The relationship between CFAE and arrhythmogenic substrates has been reported in recent studies [61, 82, 87, 50, 49, 119–121]. However, how to differentiate the fragmented EGM according to the substrate that generates it? It has been observed that the *ApEn* maps, calculated from the standard parameters (*ApEn* (2, 0.1, 500) and *ApEn* (2, 0.1, 1000)), present fragmentation with high *ApEn* levels for the rotors R1 and R2, for the blockade at right inferior pulmonary vein and the coronary sinus region; however, they do not present significant numerical differences. This has also been observed by Navoret et al. [88], who establish a relationship between detected

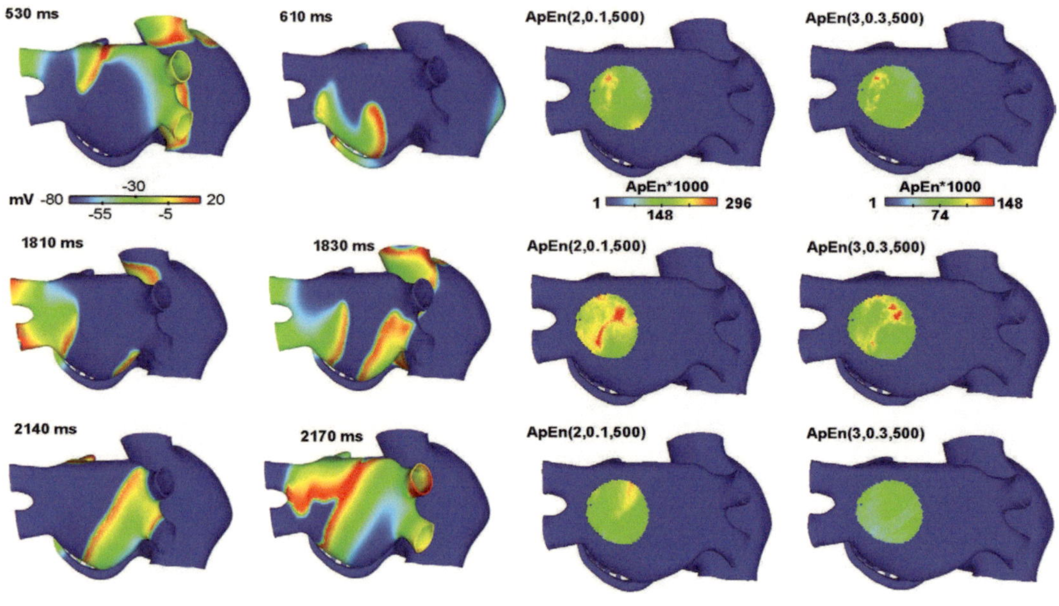

Figure 10. Three consecutive frames of propagation (first and second columns) of a meandering rotor and the Pincus parameters ApEn map (third column) and optimized parameters ApEn map (fourth column).

CFAE and the presence of wave and rotor shock, but they cannot differentiate them, using two-dimensional computational models and cell cultures. They also report the development of an algorithm, which extracts five characteristics for the characterization of fragmented EGM. The algorithm is tested in two real databases: the first has EGM labeled as fragmented and nonfragmented. The algorithm shows good results in the classification. The second has EGM labeled as active fragmentation, whose ablation restored sinus rhythm, and fragmentation whose ablation did not restore sinus rhythm. The algorithm did not discriminate between both classifications [48]. However, the *ApEn* maps, calculated using the optimized parameters optimized (*ApEn*(3, 0.3, 500) and *ApEn*(3, 0.38, 1000)), assign values by ranges to areas of interest, the R1 and R2 rotors being the highest *ApEn*, followed by the intermediate values of *ApEn* in the zone of the blockade and the coronary sinus, and the smaller values of *ApEn* to the fibrillatory EGM of regular morphology. These results suggest that: the *ApEn* can solve the problem described by Navoret et al. [88]. On the other hand, if it is verified that the ablation guided by the *ApEn* maps restores the sinus rhythm, it solves the problem reported in Ref. [28]. Future work should focus on evaluating, in computational and experimental models, ablation guided by maps of dynamic *ApEn*.

Some authors have pointed out the disadvantages of *ApEn*: it is not a stable measure when the number of points N varies, and it has an inherent deviation from the real value, due to the inclusion of self-comparison of segments [122, 123]. It has even been proposed a new statistical, the sample entropy (*SampEn*), as an enhancement of the *ApEn* [97]. However, it has been shown that both have a same behavior for time series of fast dynamics [110, 114, 124]. In our research, the possible instability that can present the *ApEn* due to the variation of points does not influence the results: specific families of *ApEn* have been defined, starting from the election of the r y m parameters, using time series of 500 and 1000 points. Although it has been observed that the range of *ApEn* values varies for each case, the information provided by the *ApEn* is embedded in the continuous scale that it results, given the degrees of irregularity that the fibrillatory EGM may present. This feature is important, since it offers adaptability to the wide range of EGM morphologies that may present different cases. In addition, it is not necessary to define intervals of fixed *ApEn* values for CFAE identification. It is only necessary to define that the *ApEn* scale, during an AF episode, is proportional to the presence of fragmentation, where the higher values of *ApEn* suggest the presence of rotors.

5.2. Multifractal analysis of EGM signals

Fluctuations in EGM signals are nonperiodic and exhibit nonlinear behavior. Fractal models could be used to describe this behavior through the identification of self-similarity and scale invariance in the statistical properties of the signals. Fractal signals present self-similarities and scale invariance properties that can be described by a single quantity, for example, the Hausdorff dimension or the Hurst exponent, and it is represented using a power law relationship. Fractal properties of physiological signals are not homogeneous, which means that local scaling properties change with time, and there is necessary to use different local Hurts exponent to describe the evolution of the system. Therefore, multifractal analysis could capture these changes in the global singularity distributions [101]. Then, the power law for multifractal behavior is written as follows:

$$N_{\alpha} \sim \epsilon^{-f(\alpha)} \tag{4}$$

where N_{α} corresponds to the number of balls with a singular exponent equal to some value of α, necessary to cover a specific set, ϵ is the diameter of the balls that covered the set, and $f(\alpha)$ corresponds to the Hausdorff dimension. Note that in fractal analysis, the exponent is a scalar, while here the exponent is a function that contain different local Hurts exponent.

To compute the singular spectrum $f(\alpha)$, we used a method called multifractal detrended fluctuation analysis proposed and described in Ref. [125]. Using $f(\alpha)$, we calculate the h-fluctuation index as is described by Orozco-Duque et al. [101].

5.3. Location of simulated rotors using multifractal analysis

Multifractal analysis can be used to calculate features such as h-fluctuation index and to build electroanatomical maps to located sites fractal or multifractal activity. This measure is related to the complexity of the EGM signals recorded over the atrial surface. In this case, we work with signals recorded from a simulated episode of AF in the three-dimensional model described above. **Figure 11A** shows a color map built with the values obtained by the multifractal analysis according with Orozco-Duque et al. [126]. Here, red dots are locating in regions where the rotor tip is presented in the model, and in the neighborhood of the rotor tip where the tip is meandering.

On the other hand, h-fluctuation index was calculated in EGM signals recorded from the two-dimensional simulated episode of fibrillatory conduction. For the sake of comparison, *ApEn* map was computed using the two-dimensional model and the optimized parameters.

These features were calculated for each EGM individually, and values were represented in a color map. **Figure 11B** shows the *ApEn* map and **Figure 5** represented the MF map. *ApEn* map exhibits the behavior of the rotor tip and illustrates the dynamics in the vicinity of the pivot point. In the central point of the rotor, there is a blue point representing some organized signals; however, in the neighborhood of the tip, there are reds dots that represent signals with high fragmented activity. A start-shaped pattern can be identified, which represents the movement of the singularity point.

In **Figure 11C**, multifractal map exhibits an interesting behavior because it captures the dynamic of the whole rotor in the atrial tissue, not only the neighborhood of the tip. One can note that the direction of the rotation is illustrated and can be interpreted using this map.

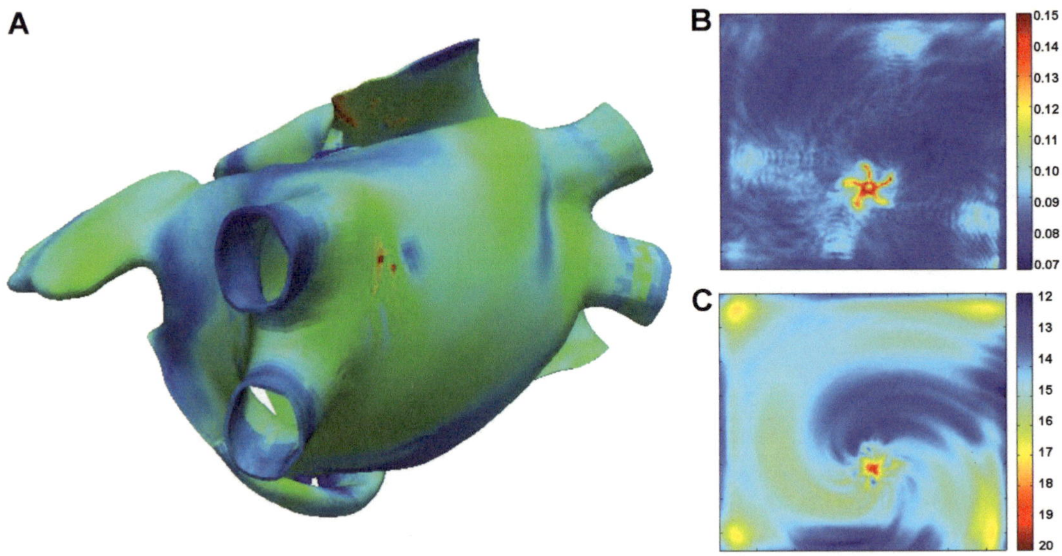

Figure 11. (A) Three-dimensional electroanatomical map using multifractal analysis. (B) Two-dimensional electroanatomical map using ApEn. (C) Two-dimensional electroanatomical map using multifractal analysis.

6. Combination of features in the same EA map

EGM signals exhibit different morphologies that have not been enough studied. An inadequate characterization of EGM morphologies has limited the success of EGM-guide ablation strategies. Looking for a better description of different EGM patterns, some authors have proposed the combination of features to detect critical sites in AF. This approach has the advantage of use different information from the signals and detects patterns that could be associated with wave collisions, conduction block, or pivot points.

Ravelli et al. [127] used a logical digital map to combined two indexes, one based on the detection of activation rate, the cycle length; and another based on the analysis of similarities between activation waves, the similarity (S). Logical operator map can discriminate two morphologies: rapidly organized and rapidly fragmented. According with Kalifa et al. rapidly organized, EGM could be associated with localized source of AF, while rapidly fragmented could be associated with the neighborhood of a pivot point [52]. One limitation of the approach proposed by Ravelli et al. is that the computation of cycle length and S requires the segmentation of EGM signals and the detection of local activation waves (LAW). This process is not always feasible especially with high-disorganized patterns.

Schilling et al. proposed an approach based on a classifier called Fuzzy decision tree to combine features and classify the EGM signals among four classes [128]. Classes are assigned according to a modified Well's criteria, where class 0 corresponds to organized and nonfragmented signal, class 1 is assigned to signals with fragmented waves but periodic activity, class 2 corresponds to signals with fragmented waves with periodic and nonperiodic activity, and class 3 is assigned to signals with high frequency and continuous activity. A limitation for using supervised learning is that the classifier depends on the classes selected by the group who collected the training database. This could be critical and bias the results because there is not a complete understanding about EGM morphologies.

Unsupervised learning has been proposed to combine features and creates maps to show the distribution of EGM cluster according with conduction patterns. We have tested some clustering methods based on machine learning such as K-means and Self-Organized Maps (SOM) in previous work. To locate rotors over simulation in two-dimensional models, the best performance was obtained using the combination of Shannon Entropy and the mean value of the EGM signal as an input of K-means algorithm with three clusters or the SOM algorithm with four clusters. **Figure 12B** and **C** shows the result of K-means and SOM applied to signals from the two-dimensional model. The classifiers performance was calculated using the distance between the rotor tip location and the mean of the points grouped by the nearest cluster. These results evince the capability of the combination of simple features using unsupervised algorithms for rotor tip location.

The issues related to the clustering approach are the selection of clusters number and the classification of clusters to identify the set of EGM related to a specific pattern. To overcome these limitations, Orozco-Duque et al. [129] have proposed a semisupervised clustering approach to combine features. Semisupervised clustering (SC) is not limited to previously defined classes. The method selected was spectral clustering with an automatic detection of cluster number. In a previous work, it was tested the performance of SC to discriminated between four classes according with the scheme proposed by Schilling et al. [130]. We tested SC and its feasibility to located pivot points in simulated episodes of AF. We used unipolar signals acquired in an AF simulation using the three-dimensional model of human atrial. **Figure 12A** shows a map built from the results of SC evaluation. Four clusters were detected; the cluster that represents regular signals is displayed in blue, and the cluster with the highest disorganized pattern is displayed in red. This cluster is located in the areas where the two rotors meander. The distribution of yellow and green clusters gives us an idea about cluster rotation.

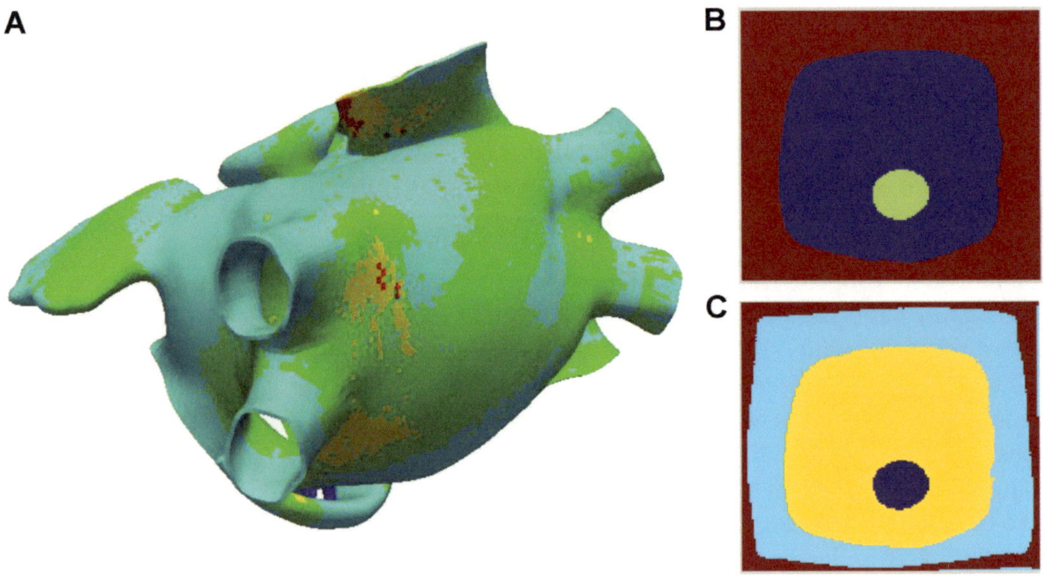

Figure 12. (A) Electroanatomical map using semisupervised clustering applied to signals from three-dimensional model. (B) Two-dimensional electroanatomical map using K-means. (C) Electroanatomical map using SOM.

7. Concluding remarks

Phase maps are, currently, the accepted tools for rotor characterization [131], by tracking the tip through the phase singularity. Although it is widely applied in computational studies [132, 133] and in vitro experimentation, such as optical mapping [134, 135], clinical application presents technical limitations: high spatial resolution and EGM require a preprocessing stage in which information of activation can be lost [136]. Here, we have presented how nonlinear features and clustering approaches provide information about the rotor dynamics during AF virtual episodes. Translated to a clinical context, these measures can be extracted from real EGM without needing special signal conditioning. However, our simulations provide high spatial resolution that places the same limitation as phase maps. In a recent report [137], we tested the influence of the spatial resolution over the *ApEn* electroanatomical maps in detecting rotors, using a two-dimensional atrial fibrillation model. Our results indicate that the *ApEn* maps can identify the rotor tip with spatial resolutions close to those available in commercial mapping catheters. We also showed that a minor dependence of the *ApEn* maps on the virtual electrode array position, which implies that there is a transition of irregularity starting at the rotor tip and spreading to its surroundings. These findings encourage considering nonlinear features for EGM analysis. Although experimental validation is needed, further in silico studies are needed to enhance and characterize the behavior of these tools.

Nonlinear features such as *ApEn* and indexes calculated from multifractal analysis allow the construction of maps to display the distribution of EGM morphologies and to study the

http://dx.doi.org/10.5772/intechopen.69475

dynamic of fibrillatory conduction in the atrial surface. Additionally, application of clustering tools allows us to incorporate the information from different features within the same system for study the distribution of EGM clusters in the atrial surface. The use of unsupervised learning approach has the vantage that does not depend on a training specific dataset, which is an important feature considering the gaps in the knowledge about EGM morphologies. In AF simulated models, rotors were located by the proposed methodology; however, further observations and clinical studies are needed to associate marked sites with arrhythmogenic substrates in humans.

Author details

Catalina Tobón[1], Andrés Orozco-Duque[2], Juan P. Ugarte[3], Miguel Becerra[4*] and Javier Saiz[5]

*Address all correspondence to: migb2b@gmail.com

1 MATBIOM, Universidad de Medellín, Medellín, Colombia

2 GI^{2}B, Instituto Tecnológico Metropolitano, Medellín, Colombia

3 Centro de Bioingeniería, Universidad Pontificia Bolivariana, Medellín, Colombia

4 Institución Universitaria Salazar y Herrera, Medellín, Colombia

5 CI^{2}B, Universitat Politècnica de València, Valencia, España

References

[1] Wolf PA, Benhamin EJ, Belanger AJ, Kannel WB, Levy D, D'Agostino RB. Secular trends in the prevalence of atrial fibrillation: The Framingham study. American Heart Journal. 1996;**131**(4):790-795

[2] MiyasakaY, Barnes ME, Gersh BJ, Cha SS, Seward JB, Bailey KR, Iwasaka T, Tsang TSM. Time trends of ischemic stroke incidence and mortality in patients diagnosed with first atrial fibrillation in 1980-2000: Report of a community-based study. Stroke. 2005;**36**(11):2362-2366

[3] Fuster V, Rydén LE, Cannom DS, Crijns HJ, Curtis AB, Ellenbogen KA, Halperin JL, Le Heuzey J, Kay GN, Lowe JE, Olsson SB, Prystowsky EN, Tamargo JL, Aha ACC, Force T, Smith SC, Jacobs AK, Adams CD, Anderson JL, Antman EM, Hunt SA, Nishimura R, Ornato JP, Page RL, Committee ESC, Practice FOR, Priori SG, Blanc J, Budaj A, Camm AJ, Dean V, Deckers JW, Morais J, Osterspey A, Zamorano JL. ACC/AHA/ESC 2006 guidelines for the management of patients with atrial fibrillation. Circulation. 2006;**114**(7):700-752

[4] Kannel WB, Wolf PA, Benjamin EJ, Levy D. Prevalence, incidence, prognosis, and predisposing conditions for atrial fibrillation: Population-based estimates. American Journal of Cardiology. 1998;**82**(8A):2N-9N

[5] Nattel S. New ideas about atrial fibrillation 50 years on. Nature. 2002;**415**(6868):219-226

[6] Voigt N, Maguy A, Yeh YH, Qi X, Ravens U, Dobrev D, Nattel S. Changes in IK, ACh single-channel activity with atrial tachycardia remodelling in canine atrial cardiomyocytes. Cardiovascular Research. 2008;**77**(1):35-43

[7] Ausma J, Van der Velden HMW, Lenders MH, Van Ankeren EP, Jongsma HJ, Ramaekers FCS, Borgers M, Allessie MA. Reverse structural and gap-junctional remodeling after prolonged atrial fibrillation in the goat. Circulation. 2003;**107**(15):2051-2058

[8] Wijffels MC, Kirchhof CJ, Dorland R, Allessie MA. Atrial fibrillation begets atrial fibrillation. A study in awake chronically instrumented goats. Circulation. 1995;**92**(7):1954-1968

[9] Workman AJ, Kane KA, Rankin AC. The contribution of ionic currents to changes in refractoriness of human atrial myocytes associated with chronic atrial fibrillation. Cardiovascular Research. 2001;**52**(2):226-235

[10] Bosch RF, Zeng X, Grammer JB, Popovic K, Mewis C, Kühlkamp V. Ionic mechanisms of electrical remodeling in human atrial fibrillation. Cardiovascular Research. 1999;**44**(1):121-131

[11] Nattel S, Burstein B, Dobrev D. Atrial remodeling and atrial fibrillation: Mechanisms and implications. Circulation. Arrhythmia and Electrophysiology. 2008;**1**(1):62-73

[12] Allessie MA. Atrial electrophysiologic remodeling: Another vicious circle? Journal of Cardiovascular Electrophysiology. 1998;**9**(12):1378-1393

[13] HaissaguerreM, Jais P, Shah DC, Takahashi A, Hocini M, Quiniou G, Garrigue S, Le Mouroux A, Le Métayer P, Clémenty J. Spontaneous initiation of atrial fibrillation by ectopic beats originating in the pulmonary veins. The New England Journal of Medicine. 1998;**339**(10):659-666

[14] Mandapati R, Skanes A, Chen J, Berenfeld O, Jalife J. Stable microreentrant sources as a mechanism of atrial fibrillation in the isolated sheep heart. Circulation. 2000;**101**(2):194-199

[15] JalifeJ. Rotors and spiral waves in atrial fibrillation. Journal of Cardiovascular Electrophysiology. 2003;**14**(7):776-780

[16] Chen SA, Hsieh MH, Tai CT, Tsai CF, Prakash VS, Yu WC, Hsu TL, Ding YA, Chang MS. Initiation of atrial fibrillation by ectopic beats originating from the pulmonary veins: Electrophysiological characteristics, pharmacological responses, and effects of radiofrequency ablation. Circulation. 1999;**100**(18):1879-1886

[17] Chen YJ, Chen SA, Chang MS, Lin CI. Arrhythmogenic activity of cardiac muscle in pulmonary veins of the dog: Implication for the genesis of atrial fibrillation. Cardiovascular Research. 2000;**48**(2):265-273

[18] Veenhuyzen GD, Simpson CS, Abdollah H. Atrial fibrillation. Canadian Medical Association Journal. 2004;**171**(7):755-760

[19] Weiss JN, Qu Z, Shivkumar K. Ablating atrial fibrillation: A translational science perspective for clinicians. Heart Rhythm. 2016;**13**(9):1868-1877

[20] de Vos CB, Pisters R, Nieuwlaat R, Prins MH, Tieleman RG, Coelen RJS, van den Heijkant AC, Allessie MA, Crijns HJGM. Progression from paroxysmal to persistent atrial fibrillation. Clinical Correlates and Prognosis. Journal of the American College of Cardiology. 2010;**55**(8):725-731

[21] De Groot NMS, Schalij MJ. Fragmented, long-duration, low-amplitude electrograms characterize the origin of focal atrial tachycardia. Journal of Cardiovascular Electrophysiology. 2006;**17**(10):1086-1092

[22] Pison L, Tilz R, Jalife J, Haissaguerre M. Pulmonary vein triggers, focal sources, rotors and atrial cardiomyopathy: Implications for the choice of the most effective ablation therapy. Journal of Internal Medicine. 2016;**279**(5):449-456

[23] Sanders P, Berenfeld O, Hocini M, Jaïs P, Vaidyanathan R, Hsu L-F, Garrigue S, Takahashi Y, Rotter M, Sacher F, Scavée C, Ploutz-Snyder R, Jalife J, Haïssaguerre M. Spectral analysis identifies sites of high-frequency activity maintaining atrial fibrillation in humans. Circulation. 2005;**112**(6):789-797

[24] Narayan SM, Krummen DE, Shivkumar K, Clopton P, Rappel WJ, Miller JM. Treatment of atrial fibrillation by the ablation of localized sources. Journal of the American College of Cardiology. 2012;**60**(7):628-636

[25] Hansen BJ, Zhao J, Csepe TA, Moore BT, Li N, Jayne LA, Kalyanasundaram A, Lim P, Bratasz A, Powell KA, Simonetti OP, Higgins RSD, Kilic A, Mohler P, Janssen JPML, Weiss R, Hummel JD, Fedorov VV. Atrial fibrillation driven by micro-anatomic intramural re-entry revealed by simultaneous sub-epicardial and sub-endocardial optical mapping in explanted human hearts. European Heart Journal. 2015;**36**(35):2390-2401

[26] Mansour M, Mandapati R, Berenfeld O, Chen J, Samie FH, Jalife J. Left-to-right gradient of atrial frequencies during acute atrial fibrillation in the isolated sheep heart. Circulation. 2001;**103**(21):2631-2636

[27] Jalife J, Berenfeld O, Mansour M. Mother rotors and fibrillatory conduction: A mechanism of atrial fibrillation. Cardiovascular Research. 2002;**54**(2):204-216

[28] Climent AM, Guillem MS, Fuentes L, Lee P, Bollensdorff C, Fernandez-Santos ME, Suarez-Sancho S, Sanz-Ruiz R, Sanchez PL, Atienza F, Fernandez-Aviles F. The role of atrial tissue remodeling on rotor dynamics: An in-vitro study. The American Journal of Physiology-Heart and Circulatory Physiology. 2015;**309**:H1964-H1973

[29] Skanes AC, Mandapati R, Berenfeld O, Davidenko JM, Jalife J. Spatiotemporal periodicity during atrial fibrillation in the isolated sheep heart. Circulation. 1998;**98**(12):1236-1248

[30] Wieser L, Nowak CN, Tilg B, Fischer G. Mother rotor anchoring in branching tissue with heterogeneous membrane properties. Biomedical Technician Education. 2008;**53**(1):25-35

[31] Narayan SM, Krummen DE, Rappel WJ. Clinical mapping approach to diagnose electrical rotors and focal impulse sources for human atrial fibrillation, Journal of Cardiovascular Electrophysiology. 2012;**23**(5):447-454

[32] Haissaguerre M, Hocini M, Denis A, Shah AJ, Komatsu Y, Yamashita S, Daly M, Amraoui S, Zellerhoff S, Picat MQ, Quotb A, Jesel L, Lim H, Ploux S, Bordachar P, Attuel G, Meillet V, Ritter P, Derval N, Sacher F, Bernus O, Cochet H, Jais P, Dubois R. Driver domains in persistent atrial fibrillation. Circulation. 2014;**130**(7):530-538

[33] Narayan SM, Patel J, Mulpuru S, Krummen DE. Focal impulse and rotor modulation ablation of sustaining rotors abruptly terminates persistent atrial fibrillation to sinus rhythm with elimination of follow-up: A video case study. Heart Rhythm. 2012;**9**(9):1436-1439

[34] Narayan SM, Shivkumar K, Krummen DE, Miller JM, Rappel WJ. Panoramic electrophysiological mapping but not electrogram morphology identifies stable sources for human atrial fibrillation: Stable atrial fibrillation rotors and focal sources relate poorly to fractionated electrograms. Circulation: Arrhythmia and Electrophysiology. 2013;**6**(1):58-67

[35] Reumann M, Bohnert J, Osswald B, Hagl S, Doessel O. Multiple wavelets, rotors, and snakes in atrial fibrillation-a computer simulation study. Journal of Electrocardiology. 2007;**40**(4):328-334

[36] UgarteJ P, Orozco-Duque ACTN, Kremen V, Novak D, Saiz J, Oesterlein T, Schmitt C, Luik A, Bustamante J. Dynamic approximate entropy electroanatomic maps detect rotors in a simulated atrial fibrillation model. PLoS One. 2014;**9**(12):e114577.

[37] Calvo CJ, Deo M, Zlochiver S, Millet J, Berenfeld O. Attraction of rotors to the pulmonary veins in paroxysmal atrial fibrillation: A modeling study. Biophysical Journal. 2014;**106**(8):1811-1821

[38] Gonzales MJ, Vincent KP, Rappel WJ, Narayan SM, McCulloch AD. Structural contributions to fibrillatory rotors in a patient-derived computational model of the atria. Europace. 2014;**16**:iv3-iv10

[39] Nademanee K, Lockwood E, Oketani N, Gidney B. Catheter ablation of atrial fibrillation guided by complex fractionated atrial electrogram mapping of atrial fibrillation substrate. Journal of Cardiology. 2010;**55**(1):1-12

[40] January CT, Wann LS, Alpert JS, Calkins H, Cigarroa JE, Cleveland JC, Conti JB, Ellinor PT, Ezekowitz MD, Field ME, Murray KT, Sacco RL, Stevenson WG, Tchou PJ, Tracy CM, Yancy CW. 2014 AHA/ACC/HRS guideline for the management of patients with atrial fibrillation. Journal of the American College of Cardiology. 2014;**64**(21):e1-e76

[41] Bhargava M, Di Biase L, Mohanty P, Prasad S, Martin DO, Williams-Andrews M, Wazni OM, Burkhardt JD, Cummings JE, Khaykin Y, Verma A, Hao S, Beheiry S, Hongo R, Rossillo A, Raviele A, Bonso A, Themistoclakis S, Stewart K, Saliba WI, Schweikert RA, Natale A.

Impact of type of atrial fibrillation and repeat catheter ablation on long-term freedom from atrial fibrillation: Results from a multicenter study. Heart Rhythm. 2009;**6**(10):1403-1412

[42] TobónC, Ruiz-Villa CA, Heidenreich E, Romero L, Hornero F, Saiz J. A three-dimensional human atrial model with fiber orientation. Electrograms and arrhythmic activation patterns relationship. PLoS One. 2013;**8**(2):e50883

[43] Song JS, Lee YS, Hwang M, Lee JK, Li C, Joung B, Lee MH, Shim EB, Pak HN. Spatial reproducibility of complex fractionated atrial electrogram depending on the direction and configuration of bipolar electrodes: An in-silico modeling study. Korean Journal of Physiology and Pharmacology. 2016;**20**(5):507-514

[44] Jacquemet V, Virag N, Ihara Z, Dang L, Blanc O, Zozor S, Vesin JM, Kappenberger L, Henriquez CS. Study of unipolar electrogram morphology in a computer model of atrial fibrillation. Journal of Cardiovascular Electrophysiology. 2003;**14**(10 Suppl):S172-S179

[45] Zlochiver S, Yamazaki M, Kalifa J, Berenfeld O. Rotor meandering contributes to irregularity in electrograms during atrial fibrillation. Heart Rhythm. 2008;**5**(6):846-854

[46] Nademanee K, McKenzie J, Kosar E, Schwab M, Sunsaneewitayakul B, Vasavakul T, Khunnawat C, Ngarmukos T. A new approach for catheter ablation of atrial fibrillation: Mapping of the electrophysiologic substrate. Journal of the American College of Cardiology. 2004;**43**(11):2044-2053

[47] Ganesan AN, Kuklik P, Lau DH, Brooks AG, Baumert M, Lim WW, Thanigaimani S, Nayyar S, Mahajan R, Kalman JM, Roberts-Thomson KC, Sanders P. Bipolar electrogram Shannon entropy at sites of rotational activation: Implications for ablation of atrial fibrillation. Circulation: Arrhythmia and Electrophysiology. 2013;**6**(1):48-57

[48] Navoret N, Jacquir S, Laurent G, Binczak S. Detection of complex fractionated atrial electrograms using recurrence quantification analysis. IEEE Transactions on Biomedical Engineering. 2013;**60**(7):1975-1982

[49] Navoret N, Jacquir S, Laurent G, Binczak S. Relationship between complex fractionated atrial electrogram patterns and different heart substrate configurations materials numerical cell models method, the modelled catheter is a thermocool irrigated tip. Computing in Cardiology. 2012;**39**:893-896

[50] Umapathy K, Masse S, Kolodziejska K, Veenhuyzen GD, Chauhan VS, Husain M, Farid T, Downar E, Sevaptsidis E, Nanthakumar K. Electrogram fractionation in murine HL-1 atrial monolayer model. Heart Rhythm. 2008;**5**(7):1029-1035

[51] Lin YJ, Tsao HM, Chang SL, Lo LW, Hu YF, Chang CJ, Tsai WC, Suenari K, Huang SY, Chang HY, Wu TJ, Chen SA. Role of high dominant frequency sites in nonparoxysmal atrial fibrillation patients: Insights from high-density frequency and fractionation mapping. Heart Rhythm. 2010;**7**(9):1255-1262

[52] Kalifa J, Tanaka K, Zaitsev AV, Warren M, Vaidyanathan R, Auerbach D, Pandit S, Vikstrom KL, Ploutz-Snyder R, Talkachou A, Atienza F, Guiraudon G, Jalife J,

Berenfeld O. Mechanisms of wave fractionation at boundaries of high-frequency excitation in the posterior left atrium of the isolated sheep heart during atrial fibrillation. Circulation. 2006;**113**(5):626-633

[53] Berenfeld O, Mandapati R, Dixit S, Skanes AC, Chen JAY, Mansour M, Jalife J. Spatially distributed dominant excitation frequencies reveal hidden organization in atrial fibrillation in the Langendorff-perfused sheep heart. Journal of Cardiovascular Electrophysiology. 2000;**11**(8):869-879

[54] Lazar S, Dixit S, Marchlinski FE, Callans DJ, Gerstenfeld EP. Presence of left-to-right atrial frequency gradient in paroxysmal but not persistent atrial fibrillation in humans. Circulation. 2004;**110**(20):3181-3186

[55] Sanders P, Nalliah CJ, Dubois R, Takahashi Y, Hocini M, Rotter M, Rostock T, Sacher F, Hsu LF, Jonsson A, O'Neill MD, Jais P, Haissaguerre M. Frequency mapping of the pulmonary veins in paroxysmal versus permanent atrial fibrillation. Journal of Cardiovascular Electrophysiology. 2006;**17**(9):965-972

[56] Oral H, Chugh A, Good E, Wimmer A, Dey S, Gadeela N, Sankaran S, Crawford T, Sarrazin JF, Kuhne M, Chalfoun N, Wells D, Frederick M, Fortino J, Benloucif-Moore S, Jongnarangsin K, Pelosi F, Bogun F, Morady F. Radiofrequency catheter ablation of chronic atrial fibrillation guided by complex electrograms. Circulation. 2007;**115**(20):2606-2612

[57] Gupta AK, Maheshwari A, Thakur R, Lokhandwala YY. Cardiac mapping: Utility or futility? Indian Pacing and Electrophysiology Journal. 2002;**2**(1):20-32

[58] Reddy VY. Atrial fibrillation: Unanswered questions and future directions. Cardiology Clinics. 2009;**27**(1):201-216

[59] Chen J, Lin Y, Chen L, Yu J, Du Z, Li S, Yang Z, Zeng C, Lai X, Lu Q, Tian B, Zhou J, Xu J, Zhang A, Li Z. A decade of complex fractionated electrograms catheter-based ablation for atrial fibrillation: Literature analysis, meta-analysis and systematic review. IJC Heart & Vessels. 2014;**4**(1):63-72

[60] Jadidi AS, Duncan E, Miyazaki S, Lellouche N, Shah AJ, Forclaz A, Nault I, Wright M, Rivard L, Liu X, Scherr D, Wilton SB, Derval N, Knecht S, Kim SJ. Functional nature of electrogram fractionation demonstrated by left atrial high-density mapping. 2012; **5**(1):32-42

[61] De Bakker JMT, Wittkampf FHM. The pathophysiologic basis of fractionated and complex electrograms and the impact of recording techniques on their detection and interpretation. Circulation: Arrhythmia and Electrophysiology. 2010;**3**(2):204-213

[62] CiaccioEJ, Biviano AB, Whang W, Garan H. Identification of recurring patterns in fractionated atrial electrograms using new transform coefficients. BioMedical Engineering OnLine. 2012;**11**(1):4

[63] Courtemanche M, Ramirez RJ, Nattel S. Ionic mechanisms underlying human atrial action potential properties: Insights from a mathematical model. The American Journal of Physiology-Heart and Circulatory Physiology. 1998;**275**:H301-H321

[64] Nygren I, Fiset C, Firek L, Clark JW, Lindblad DS, Clark RB, Giles WR. Mathematical model of an adult human atrial cell: The role of K+ currents in repolarization. Circulation Research. 1998;**82**(1):63-81

[65] Maleckar MM, Greenstein JL, Trayanova NA, Giles WR. Mathematical simulations of ligand-gated and cell-type specific effects on the action potential of human atrium. Progress in Biophysics & Molecular Biology. 2008;**98**(2-3):161-170

[66] Koivumaki JT, Korhonen T, Tavi P. Impact of sarcoplasmic reticulum calcium release on calcium dynamics and action potential morphology in human atrial myocytes: A computational study. PLoS Computational Biology. 2011;**7**(1):e1001067

[67] Grandi E, Pandit SV, Voigt N, Workman AJ, Dobrev D, Jalife J, Bers DM. Human atrial action potential and Ca^{2+} model: Sinus rhythm and chronic atrial fibrillation. Circulation Research. 2011;**109**(9):1055-1066

[68] Kneller J, Zou R, Vigmond EJ, Wang Z, Leon LJ, Nattel S. Cholinergic atrial fibrillation in a computer model of a two-dimensional sheet of canine atrial cells with realistic ionic properties. Circulation Research. 2002;**90**(9):E73–E87

[69] Van Wagoner DR. Electrophysiological remodeling in human atrial fibrillation. Pacing and Clinical Electrophysiology. 2003;**26**(7 Pt 2):1572-1575

[70] Pandit S, Berenfeld O, Anumonwo JMB, Zaritski RM, Kneller J, Nattel S, Jalife J. Ionic determinants of functional reentry in a 2-D model of human atrial cells during simulated chronic atrial fibrillation. Biophysical Journal. 2005;**88**(6):3806-3821

[71] Heidenreich EA, Ferrero JM, Doblaré M, Rodríguez JF. Adaptive macro finite elements for the numerical solution of monodomain equations in cardiac electrophysiology. Annals of Biomedical Engineering. 2010;**38**(7):2331-2345

[72] Harrild D, Henriquez C. A computer model of normal conduction in the human atria. Circulation Research. 2000;**87**(7):E25–E36

[73] Sachse FB, Frech R, Werner CD, Dossel O. A model based approach to assignment of myocardial fibre orientation. Computers in Cardiology. 1999;**26**:145-148

[74] Tobón C, Rodríguez JF, Ferrero JM, Hornero F, Saiz J. Dominant frequency and organization index maps in a realistic three-dimensional computational model of atrial fibrillation. Europace. 2012;**14**:v25-v32

[75] Seemann G, Höper C, Sachse FB, Dössel O, Holden AV, Zhang H. Heterogeneous three-dimensional anatomical and electrophysiological model of human atria. Philosophical transactions. Series A, Mathematical, Physical, and Engineering Sciences. 2006;**364**(1843):1465-1481

[76] Dang L, Virag N, Ihara Z, Jacquemet V, Vesin JM, Schlaepfer J, Ruchat P, Kappenberger L. Evaluation of ablation patterns using a biophysical model of atrial fibrillation. Annals of Biomedical Engineering. 2005;**33**(4):465-474

[77] Kharche S, Zhang H. Simulating the effects of atrial fibrillation induced electrical remodeling: a comprehensive simulation study. Conference Proceedings: IEEE Engineering in Medicine and Biology Society. 2008;**2008**:593-596

[78] Dössel O, Krueger MW, Weber FM, Wilhelms M, Seemann G. Computational modeling of the human atrial anatomy and electrophysiology. Medical & Biological Engineering & Computing. 2012;**50**(8):773-799

[79] Aslanidi OV, Colman MA, Stott J, Dobrzynski H, Boyett MR, Holden AV, Zhang H. 3D virtual human atria: A computational platform for studying clinical atrial fibrillation. Progress in Biophysics & Molecular Biology. 2011;**107**(1):156-168

[80] Zhao J, Butters TD, Zhang H, Pullan AJ, LeGrice IJ, Sands GB, Smaill BH. An image-based model of atrial muscular architecture effects of structural anisotropy on electrical activation. Circulation: Arrhythmia and Electrophysiology. 2012;**5**(2):361-370

[81] Hwang M, Song JS, Lee YS, Li C, Shim EB, Pak HN. Electrophysiological rotor ablation in in-silico modeling of atrial fibrillation: Comparisons with dominant frequency, Shannon entropy, and phase singularity. PLoS One. 2016;**11**(2):1-15

[82] Konings KT, Smeets JL, Penn OC, Wellens HJ, Allessie MA. Configuration of unipolar atrial electrograms during electrically induced atrial fibrillation in humans. Circulation. 1997;**95**(5):1231-1241

[83] Chorro FJ, Ferrero A, Canoves J, Mainar L, Porres JC, Navarro A, Sanchis J, Millet J, Bodí V, López-Merino V, Such L. Significance of the morphological patterns of electrograms recorded during ventricular fibrillation: An experimental study. PACE—Pacing and Clinical Electrophysiology. 2003;**26**(5);1262-1269

[84] Kirubakaran S, Chowdhury RA,. Hall MCS, Patel PM, Garratt CJ, Peters NS. Fractionation of electrograms is caused by colocalized conduction block and connexin disorganization in the absence of fibrosis as AF becomes persistent in the goat model. Heart Rhythm. 2015;**12**(2):397-408

[85] Ferrero JM, Ferrero JMJ, Saiz J, Arnau A. Bioelectrónica. Señales Bioeléctricas. 1994

[86] Clayton RH, Holden AV. Propagation of normal beats and re-entry in a computational model of ventricular cardiac tissue with regional differences in action potential shape and duration. Progress in Biophysics and Molecular Biology. 2004;**85**(2-3);473-499

[87] Jacquemet V, Henriquez CS. Genesis of complex fractionated atrial electrograms in zones of slow conduction: A computer model of microfibrosis. Heart Rhythm. 2009;**6**(6):803-810

[88] Navoret N, Xu B, Jacquir S, Binczak S. Comparison of complex fractionated atrial electrograms at cellular scale using numerical and experimental models. Conference Proceedings: IEEE Engineering in Medicine and Biology Society. 2010;**2010**:3249-3252

[89] Ashihara T, Haraguchi R, Nakazawa K, Namba T, Ikeda T, Nakazawa Y, Ozawa T, Ito M, Horie M, Trayanova NA. The role of fibroblasts in complex fractionated electrograms during persistent/permanent atrial fibrillation: Implications for electrogram-based catheter ablation. Circulation Research. 2012;**110**(2):275-284

[90] Yun Y, Hwang M, Park JH, Shin H, Shim EB, Pak HN. The relationship among complex fractionated electrograms, wavebreak, phase singularity, and local dominant frequency in fibrillation wave-dynamics: A modeling comparison study. Journal of Korean Medical Science. 2014;**29**(3):370-377

[91] Verma A, Sanders P, Macle L, Deisenhofer I, Morillo CA, Chen J, Jiang C, Ernst S, Mantovan R. Substrate and trigger ablation for reduction of a trial fibrillation trial-part II (STAR AF II): Design and rationale. American Heart Journal. 2012;**164**(1):1-6.e6

[92] Vogler J, Willems S, Sultan A, Schreiber D, Lüker J, Servatius H, Schäffer B, Moser J, Hoffmann BA, Steven D. Pulmonary vein isolation versus defragmentation the CHASE-AF clinical trial. Journal of the American College of Cardiology. 2015;**66**(24);2743-2752

[93] LinYJ, Lo MT, Lin C, Chang SL, Lo LW, Hu YF, Hsieh WH, Chang HY, Lin WY, Chung FP, Liao JN, Chen YY, Hanafy D, Huang NE, Chen SA. Prevalence, characteristics, mapping, and catheter ablation of potential rotors in nonparoxysmal atrial fibrillation. Circulation: Arrhythmia and Electrophysiology. 2013;**6**(5):851-858

[94] Novák D, Kremen V, Cuesta D, Schmidt K, Chudácek V, Lhotská L. Discrimination of endocardial electrogram disorganization using a signal regularity analysis. Conference Proceedings: IEEE Engineering in Medicine and Biology Society. 2009;(**2009**):1812-1815

[95] Kinsner W, Chen H. Estimating multifractal measures. In Proceedings of 1996 Canadian Conference on Electrical and Computer Engineering. 1996. pp. 716-719

[96] Pincus SM. Approximate entropy as a measure of system complexity. Proceedings of the National Academy of Sciences of the United States of America. 1991;**88**(6):2297-2301

[97] Lake DE. Improved entropy rate estimation in physiological data. Conference Proceedings: IEEE Engineering in Medicine and Biology Society. 2011;(**2011**):1463-1466

[98] Chen W, Wang Z, Xie H, Yu W. Characterization of surface EMG signal based on fuzzy entropy. IEEE Transactions on Neural Systems and Rehabilitation Engineering. 2007;**15**(2):266-272

[99] Jiang Y, Peng CK, Xu Y. Hierarchical entropy analysis for biological signals. Journal of Computational and Applied Mathematics. 2011;**236**(5):728-742

[100] Ugarte J, Orozco-Duque A, Tobón C, Kremen V, Novak D. Dynamic approximate entropy electroanatomic maps detect rotors in a simulated atrial fibrillation model. PLoS One. 2014;1-19

[101] Orozco-Duque A, Novak D, Kremen V, Bustamante J. Multifractal analysis for grading complex fractionated electrograms in atrial fibrillation. Physiological Measurement. 2015;**36**(11):2269-2284

[102] Murillo-Escobar J, Becerra MA, Cardona EA, Tobón C, Palacio LC, Valdés BE, Orrego DA. Reconstruction of Multi Spatial Resolution Feature Maps on a 2D Model of Atrial Fibrillation: Simulation Study. IFMBE proceedings. 2015;**49**:623-626

[103] Chen FW, Liu CW. Estimation of the spatial rainfall distribution using inverse distance weighting (IDW) in the middle of Taiwan. Paddy and Water Environment. 2012;**10**(3):209-222

[104] Vijayarajan R, Muttan S. Influence of iterative relaxed median filter over FCM clustering in MR images. India Conference (INDICON). 2011. pp. 1-4

[105] Babaee A, Shahrtash SM, Najafipour A. Comparing the trustworthiness of signal-to-noise ratio and peak signal-to-noise ratio in processing noisy partial discharge signals. IET Science, Measurement & Technology. 2013;**7**(2):112-118

[106] Mohktar MS, Ibrahim F, Ismail NA. Non-invasive approach to predict the cholesterol level in blood using bioimpedance and neural network techniques. 2013;**25**(6):1-7

[107] Kipli K, Muhammad MS, Masniah S, Masra W. Performance of Levenberg-Marquardt backpropagation for full reference hybrid image quality metrics. 2012;**I**:14-17

[108] Hassan M, Terrien J, Marque C, Karlsson B. Comparison between approximate entropy, correntropy and time reversibility: Application to uterine electromyogram signals. Medical Engineering Physics. 2011;**33**(8):980-986

[109] Ning X, Xu Y, Wang J, Ma X. Approximate entropy analysis of short-term HFECG based on wave mode. Physica A: Statistical Mechanics and its Applications. 2005;**346**(3-4):475-483

[110] Rigoldi C, Cimolin V, Camerota F, Celletti C, Albertini G, Mainardi L, Galli M. Measuring regularity of human postural sway using approximate entropy and sample entropy in patients with Ehlers-Danlos syndrome hypermobility type. Research in Developmental Disabilities. 2013;**34**(2):840-846

[111] Valenza G, Allegrini P, Lanatà A, Scilingo EP. Dominant lyapunov exponent and approximate entropy in heart rate variability during emotional visual elicitation. Frontiers in Neuroengineering. 2012;**5**(February):3

[112] Wu HT, Liu CC, Lo MT, Hsu PC, Liu AB, Chang KY, Tang CJ. Multiscale cross-approximate entropy analysis as a measure of complexity among the aged and diabetic. Computational and Mathematical Methods in Medicine. 2013:324325

[113] Pincus S, Singer BH. Randomness and degrees of irregularity. Proceedings of the National Academy of Sciences of the United States of America. 1996;**93**(5):2083-2088

[114] Molina-Picó A, Cuesta-Frau D, Aboy M, Crespo C, Miró-Martínez P, Oltra-Crespo S. Comparative study of approximate entropy and sample entropy robustness to spikes. Artificial Intelligence in Medicine. 2011;**53**(2):97-106

[115] Ugarte J, Orozco-Duque A, Tobón C, Kremen V, Novak D, Saiz J, Oesterlein T, Schmitt C, Luik A, Bustamante J. Dynamic approximate entropy electroanatomic maps detect rotors in a simulated atrial fibrillation model. PLoS One. 2014;**9**(12):e114577

[116] Sanjiv M, Narayan M, Wright M, Derval N, Jadidi A, Forclaz A, Nault I, Miyazaki S, Sacher F, Bordachar P, Clémenty J, Jaïs P, Haïssaguerre M, Hocini M. Classifying fractionated electrograms in human atrial fibrillation using monophasic action potentials and activation mapping: Evidence for localized drivers, rate acceleration, and nonlocal signal etiologies. Heart Rhythm. 2011;**8**(2):244-253

[117] Kremen V. Automated Assessment of Endocardial Electrograms Fractionation in Human. Czech Technical University in Prague. 2008

[118] Ohara T, Ohara KJ, Cao M, Lee MH, Fishbein MC, Mandel WJP, Chen S, Karagueuzian HS. Increased wave break during ventricular fibrillation in the epicardial border zone of hearts with healed myocardial infarction. Circulation. 2001;**103**(10):1465-1472

[119] Oketani N, Ichiki H, Iriki Y, Okui H, Ryuichi M, Fuminori N, Ninomiya Y, Ishida S, Hamasaki S, Tei C. Catheter ablation of atrial fibrillation guided by complex fractionated atrial electrogram mapping with or without pulmonary vein isolation. Journal of Arrhythmia. 2012;**28**(6):311-323

[120] Zeemering S, Maesen B, Nijs J, Lau H, Granier M, Verheule S, Schotten U. Automated quantification of atrial fibrillation complexity by probabilistic electrogram analysis and fibrillation wave reconstruction. 34th Annual International Conference of the IEEE Engineering in Medicine and Biology Society. 2012. pp. 6357-6360

[121] Kim AM, Olgin JE. Microfibrosis and complex fractionated atrial electrograms. Heart Rhythm. 2009;**6**(6):811-812

[122] Alcaraz R, Rieta JJ. A review on sample entropy applications for the non-invasive analysis of atrial fibrillation electrocardiograms. Biomedical Signal Processing and Control. 2010;**5**(1):1-14

[123] Richman JS, Moorman JR. Physiological time-series analysis using approximate entropy and sample entropy. The American Journal of Physiology-Heart and Circulatory Physiology. 2000;**278**(6):H2039-H2049

[124] Zurek S, Guzik P, Pawlak S, Kosmider M, Piskorski J. On the relation between correlation dimension, approximate entropy and sample entropy parameters, and a fast algorithm for their calculation. Physica A: Statistical Mechanics and its Applications. 2012;**391**(24):6601-6610

[125] Ihlen EAF. Introduction to multifractal detrended fluctuation analysis in Matlab. Frontiers in Physiology. 2012;**3**(June):141

[126] Orozco-Duque A, Ugarte JP, Tobon C, Saiz J, Bustamante J, Gi B, Tecnol I, Val D. Approximate entropy can localize rotors, but not ectopic foci during chronic atrial fibrillation: A simulation study. Computers in Cardiology. 2010;**2013**:903-906

[127] Ravelli F, Masè M, Cristoforetti A, Marini M, Disertori M. The logical operator map identifies novel candidate markers for critical sites in patients with atrial fibrillation. Progress in Biophysics & Molecular Biology. 2014;(**115**):186-197

[128] Schilling C, Keller M, Scherr D, Oesterlein T, Haïssaguerre M, Schmitt C, Dössel O, Luik A. Fuzzy decision tree to classify complex fractionated atrial electrograms. Biomedizinische Technik. Biomedical Engineering. 2015

[129] Orozco-Duque A, Bustamante J, Castellanos-Dominguez G. Semi-supervised clustering of fractionated electrograms for electroanatomical atrial mapping. BioMedical Engineering OnLine. 2016;**15**(1):44

[130] Schilling A. Analysis of Atrial Electrograms. Karlrsruhe: KIT Scientific Publishing; 2012. p. 17

[131] Clayton RH, Nash MP. Analysis of cardiac fibrillation using phase mapping. Cardiac Electrophysiology Clinics. 2015;**7**(1):49-58

[132] McDowell KS, Zahid S, Vadakkumpadan F, Blauer J, MacLeod RS, Trayanova NA. Virtual electrophysiological study of atrial fibrillation in fibrotic remodeling. PLoS One. 2015;**10**(2):e0117110

[133] Fenton FH, Cherry EM, Hastings HM, Evans SJ. Multiple mechanisms of spiral wave breakup in a model of cardiac electrical activity. Chaos. 2002;**12**(3):852-892

[134] Bray MA, Lin SF, Aliev RR, Roth BJ, Wikswo JP. Experimental and theoretical analysis of phase singularity dynamics in cardiac tissue. Journal of Cardiovascular Electrophysiology. 2001;**12**(6):716-722

[135] Attin M, Clusin WT. Basic concepts of optical mapping techniques in cardiac electrophysiology. Biological Research for Nursing. 2009;**11**(2):195-207

[136] Nash MP, Mourad A, Clayton RH, Sutton PM, Bradley CP, Hayward M, Paterson DJ, Taggart P. Evidence for multiple mechanisms in human ventricular fibrillation. Circulation. 2006;**114**(6):536-542

[137] Ugarte JP, Tobón C, Orozco-Duque A, Becerra MA, Bustamante J. Effect of the electrograms density in detecting and ablating the tip of the rotor during chronic atrial fibrillation: An in silico study. Europace. 2015;**17**:ii97-ii104

Chapter 9

Loss of Complexity of the Cardiac Bioelectrical Signal as an Expression of Patient Outcomes

Pedro Eduardo Alvarado Rubio,
Ricardo Mansilla Corona, Lizette Segura Vimbela,
Alejandro González Mora, Roberto Brugada Molina,
Cesar Augusto González López and
Laura Yavarik Alvarado Avila

Additional information is available at the end of the chapter

http://dx.doi.org/10.5772/intechopen.70144

Abstract

The loss of complexity of the cardiac bioelectrical signal, measured with tools of nonlinear dynamics (NLD), is studied in patients with very different pathologies. Two types of scenarios are studied: (a) patients who enter the critical care unit and recover from their condition; (b) severe patients whose condition worsen and finally die. It is shown that as the severity of the patients increases, the complexity of their cardiac bioelectric signal decreases. On the other hand, if patients, despite being severe, manage to recover, the cardiac bioelectric signal recovers its complexity.

Keywords: bioelectrical signal, nonlinear dynamics, complexity, variability, critical illness

1. Introduction

The application of tools of the theory of the dynamical systems to the study of physiological phenomena has a long inheritance. This starts from the original works of van der Pol and his collaborator [1, 2], passes through important contributions [3, 4], and reaches the comprehensive work by Glass and Mackey [5]. The application of these types of systems to describe the temporal evolution of the physiological phenomena has been established as a tool frequently used by researchers in this area of knowledge and is already a common place in the literature.

The initial works in the analysis of the dynamics of the cardiac rhythm showed a nonlinear dynamic (NLD) behavior. Period-doubling bifurcations, in which the period of a regular oscillation doubles, were predicted theoretically and observed experimentally in the heart cells of embryonic chickens [6]. The tools with a new mathematical approach made it possible to apply the nonlinear dynamics to basic physiological concepts, proving for the first time evidence of nonlinear behavior in the electrocardiogram (ECG) [7]. Period multiplying evidence in arterial blood pressure traces of a dog that had been injected with noradrenaline was reported in 1984 [8]. Since the original reports on ischemic heart disease and arrhythmia [9, 10], the analysis of spontaneous variations of beat-to-beat intervals (BBIs) has become an important clinical tool [11–13].

For a long time, the construction of models was based on first principles, being this the main tool for the understanding of complex physiological phenomena in theoretical models of nerve and the membrane [14, 15], among which the functioning of the heart occupies a main place. On the other hand, some studies tried to obtain information about cardiac diseases from the time series that the measuring instruments offered, although very often they were noisy and limited data [16]. Procedures have been developed for the study of ventricular fibrillation using the data of implantable defibrillators [13, 17]. It is well known that these data are often noisy and only represent the sequence of R-R intervals and is typically morphologically different from surface electrocardiogram recordings. Many signal-processing algorithms have been designed to eliminate noise from a system; however, noise (i.e., stochastic processes) is a critical component of many biological and physiological systems [18]. Given the difficulties mentioned earlier, some authors tried to use measures of complexity and entropies, as well as other techniques of the theory of nonlinear phenomena [19, 20].

The initial clinical observation of heart rate variability (HRV), observing changes in the pattern of the R-R interval, which preceded changes in the heart rate in fetal distress, was reported in 1963 [21]. Later, the first approaches of the heart rate variability analysis based on nonlinear fractal dynamics were performed in 1987 [4]. It was suggested that self-similar (fractal) scaling may underlie the 1/f-like spectra [22] seen in multiple systems (e.g., interbeat interval variability, daily neutrophil fluctuations). They proposed that this fractal scale invariance may provide a mechanism for the "constrained randomness" underlying physiological variability and adaptability. In 1988, it was reported that patients prone to high risk of sudden cardiac death showed evidence of nonlinear heart rate (HR) dynamics, including abrupt spectral changes and sustained low-frequency (LF) oscillations. After this report, it has been suggested that a loss of complex physiological variability could occur under certain pathological conditions such as reduced HR dynamics before sudden death and aging [23, 24].

Methods of NLD and fractal analysis have opened up new ways for the analysis of HRV. Although time and frequency domain methods enable the quantification of HRV on different time scales, nonlinear methods provide additional information regarding the dynamics and structure of beat-to-beat time series in various physiological and pathophysiological conditions [25]. The apparent loss of multiscale complexity in life-threatening conditions suggests a clinical importance of this multiscale complexity measure. Studies on heart rate multiscale entropy at 3 h predict hospital mortality in patients with major trauma [26]. Joint symbolic dynamics, compression entropy, fractal dimension, and approximate entropy revealed significantly reduced complexity of heart rate time series and loss of efferent vagal activity in acute schizophrenia [27, 28].

The healthy human heart rate is mainly determined by three major inputs: the sinoatrial node; and the parasympathetic and sympathetic branches of the autonomous nervous system and several autocrine, paracrine, and endocrine substances effects on it [29]. The sinoatrial node or pacemaker is responsible for the initiation of each heart beat; in the absence of other external stimuli, it is able to maintain an essentially constant interbeat interval. Experiments in which parasympathetic and sympathetic inputs are blocked reveal that the interbeat intervals are very regular and average 0.6 s. The parasympathetic fibers conduct impulses that increase the interbeat intervals. Suppression of sympathetic stimuli, while under parasympathetic regulation, can result in the increase of the interbeat interval to as much as 1.5 s. The activity of the parasympathetic system changes with external stimuli and with internal cycles. The sympathetic fibers conduct impulses that decrease the interbeat intervals. Abolition of parasympathetic influences when the sympathetic system remains active can decrease the interbeat intervals to less than 0.3 s. There are several centers of sympathetic activity which are highly sensitive to environmental influences [30, 31]. All the patients that are analyzed in this work have as a common factor a suffering of systemic repercussion that influences the dynamics of the sympathetic-parasympathetic balance and, therefore, of the heart rate. As will be seen subsequently, whatever the underlying condition, as it worsens, decreases the complexity of the cardiac bioelectrical signal, while its improvement is accompanied by an increase in the complexity of the cardiac signal. Hence, the measures of complexity of the heart electrical signals allow assessing the severity of the patient's condition, and as we will see later (**Figure 3**) they can be used as early warnings of severity episodes. This is why we focus on the observation of the complexity of the cardiac bioelectric signal.

The increasing availability of physiological data has allowed the study of long-time series with other techniques also coming from the theory of dynamical systems. The observations received from some organ of our body, as we have said before, very often are tainted of noise or are collected in an incomplete way. The signals of electrical activity of the heart are a good example of this. They are measured on the surface of the patient, in a finite number of places. The electrical signal from the heart must pass through several layers of tissues with different electrical conductivities before being measured by traditional devices. What we measure is actually a distorted *observable* of the authentic electric signal coming from the surface of the heart. Then the following question arises; how much information of the original phenomenon could be recovered from this distorted signal? Other relevant questions are how many magnitudes are necessary for a complete description of the phenomenon? In other words, what is the dimension of the attractor of the dynamical system that describes the evolution of the heart? Is there a difference between a healthy person and a sick person in the number of variables necessary to characterize their behavior? Or put in another way, is there a difference in the dimension of the attractor of the dynamical systems that describe the behavior of a healthy person and a sick person?

The Takens Embedding Theorem [32] answers these questions under certain assumptions about the recorded time series. In the following lines, we describe the theoretical framework, the fundamental results, and the techniques of valuation of the different magnitudes.

2. Mathematical theoretical framework

The most frequent problems in the study of the physiological signals of electrical type are that very often we have incomplete and deformed information of them. This is a very common problem in many branches of scientific knowledge. As far as the electrical activity of the cardiac muscle is concerned, a methodology has been developed, whose theoretical basis is found in the theory of dynamical systems. This result is known as the Takens' Embedding Theorem. This result allows us, under certain hypotheses, to answer the following questions: Is it possible to reconstruct the bioelectric dynamics of a cardiac phenomenon from incomplete information? How many variables are necessary to fully characterize this phenomenon?

Let us assume that n measurements would be necessary to fully characterize the phenomenon under study. We do not know them directly. Rather, we have a macroscopic observable g that is constructed from them:

$$g(t) = \theta(x_1(t), \ldots, x_n(t)) \tag{1}$$

Here, we assume that $x_1(t), \ldots, x_n(t)$ are the measurements necessary to characterize the system, measured at time t. The function θ is one that transforms the variables that characterize the system in the macroscopic observable to which we have access.

Almost all medical devices discreetly take samples with a certain frequency. Therefore, what in the practice we have is a time series $\{g_1, \ldots, g_T\}$, where $g_i = g(t_i)$, where very often it is assumed (as do we) that the times of measurement t_i are equally spaced in time.

The Takens Embedding Theorem basically says that under the assumption that function g is "well behaved," that is, which can be measured continuously without very sudden jumps then, there are $\tau \in R^+$ and $N \in N$ such that the set of vectors:

$$A_d = \left\{(g_i, g_{i+\tau}, \ldots, g_{i+(N-1)\tau}), i \in N\right\} \tag{2}$$

is for any practical purpose similar in its properties to the simultaneous behavior of the variables $x_1(t), \ldots, x_n(t)$. Unfortunately, the theorem does not say how τ and N should be calculated. So a wide heuristic has been developed to estimate these parameters [33]. In this task, two concepts play an important role: the mutual information function and the correlation integral.

The mutual information function can be defined as follows:

$$M(\tau) = \sum_{t=1}^{T-\tau} P(g_t, g_{t+\tau}) \ln\left[\frac{P(g_t, g_{t+\tau})}{P(g_t)P(g_{t+\tau})}\right] \tag{3}$$

This concept is closely related to the concept of Boltzmann entropy and the Shannon information [34]. It is a measure of nonlinear correlation among the values of the series $\{g_i\}$.

The values of the mutual information function can be calculated from the $\{g_1, \ldots, g_T\}$ series using appropriate software. The correct value for τ is the first local minimum of the mutual information function [15, 35]. It is well known that the mutual information function is more sensitive to correlations of data than other correlation measures [36].

The second important step is the calculation of the so-called embedding dimension N. For this, it is necessary to use a concept called integral correlation: consider now the collection of vector of the set A_d:

$$X_i = \left(g_i, g_{i+\tau}, \dots, g_{i+(N-1)\tau}\right) \tag{4}$$

the correlation integral $C_m(\varepsilon)$ is defined as

$$C_m(\varepsilon) = \binom{m}{2}^{-1} \sum_{1 \le i, j \le m} H(\|X_i - X_j\| < \varepsilon) \tag{5}$$

where H is the Heaviside function. From this concept, we can define the correlation dimension as

$$d_c = \lim_{\varepsilon \to 0} \lim_{m \to +\infty} \frac{\ln C_m(\varepsilon)}{\ln \varepsilon} \tag{6}$$

Now, the criteria for selecting the correct embedding dimension N are as follows: choose increasing embedding dimension and in each case, calculate the correlation integral. When no changes are observed in the behavior of the correlation integral with respect to increasing the embedding dimension, then a suitable dimension immersion [15, 33] will be found.

One of the advantages of this method is its robustness with respect to the noise of the signal under study. The numerical data obtained through a recording apparatus, in our case a Holter, are the basis of all the further calculations in this chapter. Despite the fine structures of the cardiac dynamics, a critical component of many biological and physiological systems [19], could be lost in conventional Holters [3], the attractor of the system is reconstructed with adequate embedding and correlation dimensions.

The entire process can be seen in **Figure 1**.

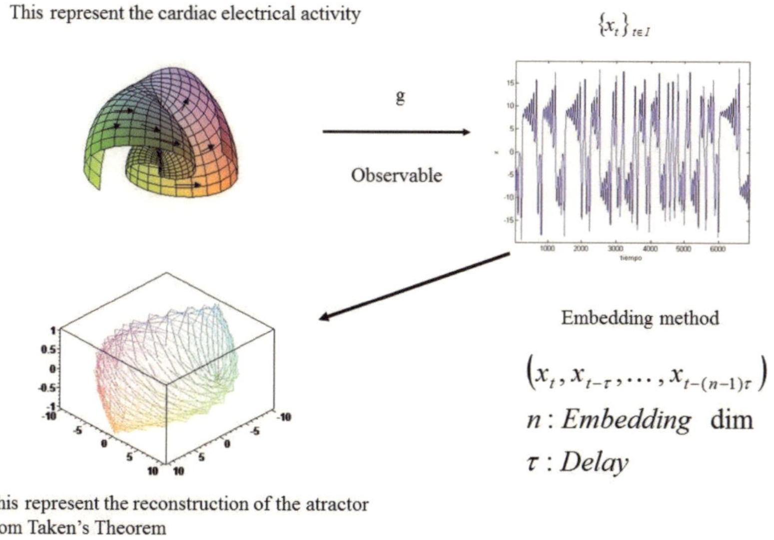

Figure 1. A representation of the entire embedding process. The phenomenon under study has an attractor which only has incomplete information through an observable. From this observable, the immersion process is executed, creating a reconstruction of the attractor.

3. Method

3.1. Description of the patients under study

We have studied the biological electrical signal of electrocardiogram assuming that its evolution is governed by a dynamic system. A three-channel, 1-h Holter (Scott Care Corporation. Chroma: Model RZ153C) Monitor was used to monitor 30 patients to obtain data files which consist of 900,000 rows and three columns of comma separated values from 1 h of registration. Holter monitoring was performed on each patient every 24 h for a period of 1 h from admission until discharge. All admission Holter records were performed with the sedated patients, with amines and ventilatory mechanical support in the supine position. The Holter records of the surviving patients also are performed in supine position, without mechanical ventilation or cardiovascular support with amines. The diagnosis of patients was performed from the clinical point of view and confirmed by imaging studies such as computed tomography (CT) of the site topologically involved, such as computed axial tomography of the skull, chest, or abdomen. Some of the patients were surgically operated on one or more occasions. We studied 30 critically ill patients (18 females, 12 male age 54.8±15.3 years old) of various pathologies, qualified with APACHE II scale 29.26 ± 3.16 on admission to intensive care.

The APACHE II Severity of Disease Classification System

Physiologic Variable	+4	+3	+2	+1	0	+1	+2	+3	+4
Temperature - rectal (°C)	≥41	39-40.9		38.5-38.9	36-38.4	34-35.9	32-33.9	30-31.9	≤29.9
Mean Arterial Pressure (mm Hg)	≥160	130-159	110-129		70-109		50-69		≤49
Heart Rate	≥180	140-179	110-139		70-109		55-69	40-54	≤39
Respiratory Rate (nonventilated or ventilated)	≥50	35-49		25-34	12-24	10-11	6-9		≤5
Oxygenation (mmHg) a. FiO_2 > 0,5 use A-aDO_2 b. FiO_2 < 0,5 use PaO_2 — a	≥500	350-499	200-349		<200				
b					> 70	61-70		55-60	<55
Arterial pH	≥7.7	7.6-7.69		7.5-7.59	7.33-7.49		7.25-7.32	7.15-7.24	<7.15
Serum Sodium (mmol/l)	≥180	160-179	155-159	150-154	130-149		120-129	111-119	≤110
Serum Potassium (mmol/l)	≥7	6-6.9		5.5-5.9	3.5-5.4	3-3.4	2.5-2.9		<2.5
Serum Creatinine (mg/dl, Double point score for acute renal failure)	≥3.5	2-3.4	1.5-1.9		0.6-1.4		<0.6		
Hematocrit (%)	≥60		50-59.9	46-49.9	30-45.9		20-29.9		<20
White Blood Count (in 1000/mm³)	≥40		20-39.9	15-19.9	3-14.9		1-2.9		<1
Glasgow-Coma-Scale (GCS)	Score = 15 minus actual GCS								
Serum HCO_3 (venous, mmol/l, use if no ABGs)	≥52	41-51.9		32-40.9	22-31.9		18-21.9	15-17.9	<15
A = Total Acute Physiology Score APS	Sum of the 12 individual variable points								
B = Age Points ≤44 years 0 points 45-54 years 2 points 55-64 years 3 points 65-74 years 5 points ≥75 years 6 points	C = Chronic Health Points If the patient has a history of severe organ system insufficiency or is immunocompromised assign points as follows: a. For nonoperative or emergency postoperative patients – 5 points b. For elective postoperative patients – 2 points								
APACHE II Score = Sum of A (APS points) + B (Age points) + C (Chronic Health points)									

(From: Knaus WA, Draper EA, Wagner DP, Zimmerman JE. APACHE II: a severity of disease classification system. Crit Care Med 1985;13(10):818-29)

The vital signs on the admission of these patients were as follows: Heart rate, 91.6 ±17.51; respiratory rate, 21.6 ± 6.43; mean arterial pressure, 71.4 ± 20.8; and temperature of 37.6 ± 1.3.

Seventy percent of the patients were admitted with cardiovascular support based on noradrenaline infusion and sedated with ventilatory mechanical support. The nonlinear time series [33] were obtained upon admission to intensive care in the morning every day, until their discharge for improvement or death. The numerical data obtained from the comma-separated values by means of the Holter are the data subject to analysis of each patient. The description of patients is shown in **Table 1**.

N°	Age	Sex	Diagnosis	Surgery N°	APACHE II/%	Survived/died
1	64	M	Severe post traumatic cerebral edema	Yes/1	27/55%	Died
2	55	F	Cerebral Hemorrhage Fisher IV Malformation Arterio/Venous	Yes/1	24/40%	Died
3	60	M	Necrotizing Pancreatitis	Yes/2	30/75%	Died
4	34	F	Traumatic Brain Injury—Intraparenchymal Hemorrhage	Yes/1	20/40%	Survived
5	78	F	Fisher IV Brain Hemorrhage by Ruptured Cerebral Aneurism	Yes/1	29/55%	Died
6	23	M	Wounded by gun fire in right eye	No	28/55%	Died
7	30	F	Postpartum complicated—Eclampsia and Pulmonary Embolism	Yes/1	27/55%	Survived
8	26	M	Septic shock by Appendicitis complicated	Yes/3	32/75%	Died
9	52	M	Cerebellar Infarction	Yes/1	28/55%	Died
10	52	F	Septic Shock of Abdominal Origin	Yes/4	30/75%	Died
11	34	M	Colon Necrosis and Septic Shock	Yes/3	29/55%	Survived
12	69	F	Epidural Hematoma	Yes/1	25/55%	Died
13	40	M	Atypical Pneumonia. Acquired Immune Deficiency	No	35/85%	Died
14	56	M	Septic Shock-Pneumonia	No	32/75%	Died
15	59	M	Pulmonary Embolism	No	30/75%	Died
16	78	F	Subarachnoid Hemorrhage—Aneurysm Rupture	Yes/1	29/55%	Died
17	63	M	Acute Myocardial Infarction	No	27/55%	Died
18	59	M	Pulmonary Embolism.	No	30/75%	Survived
19	47	F	Post Cardiorespiratory. Arrest Trans Surgical	Yes/1	32/75%	Died
20	74	F	Pulmonary Embolism.	No	27/55%	Died
21	62	F	Pulmonary Embolism.	No	28/55%	Died
22	62	M	Left cerebellar hemisphere infarction.	Yes/1	32/75%	Survived
23	47	F	Cerebral Hemorrhage - Broken Aneurysm	Yes/1	29/55%	Died
24	43	F	Cerebral Hemorrhage—Broken Aneurysm	Yes/1	29/55%	Died
25	73	F	Traumatic Brain Injury—Intraparenchymal Hemorrhage	Yes/1	30/75%	Died

N°	Age	Sex	Diagnosis	Surgery N°	APACHE II/%	Survived/died
26	60	F	Hemorrhage Fisher III. Flegmásia Cerulea Dolens	No	35/85%	Died
27	42	F	Hemorrhage Subarachnoid Fisher IV	Yes/1	30/75%	Died
28	62	F	Fisher IV Brain Hemorrhage	No	29/55%	Died
29	71	F	Cerebral Stroke	No	30/75%	Died
30	69	F	Traumatic Brain Injury—Intraparenchymal Hemorrhage	Yes/1	35/85%	Died
	54.8±15.3				29.2±3.16	

Table 1. Estimated mortality in critical patients according with APACHE II score.

The images show a CT scan where two images of patient No. 22 are shown of the posterior fossa of a 62-year-old man with hypertension treated with captopril 25 mg every 12 h. IMAGE "A" shows a hypodense zone of the left cerebellar hemisphere, suggesting an ischemic type lesion. IMAGE "B" shows decompressive craniotomy. The patient on day 10 of intensive care was without mechanical ventilation and interacting with the staff of the unit. As mentioned previously in the text, measures of the complexity of their cardiac signal were lower at the time of entry to the intensive care unit, which was recovered. Later, he was discharge from the critical medicine unit.

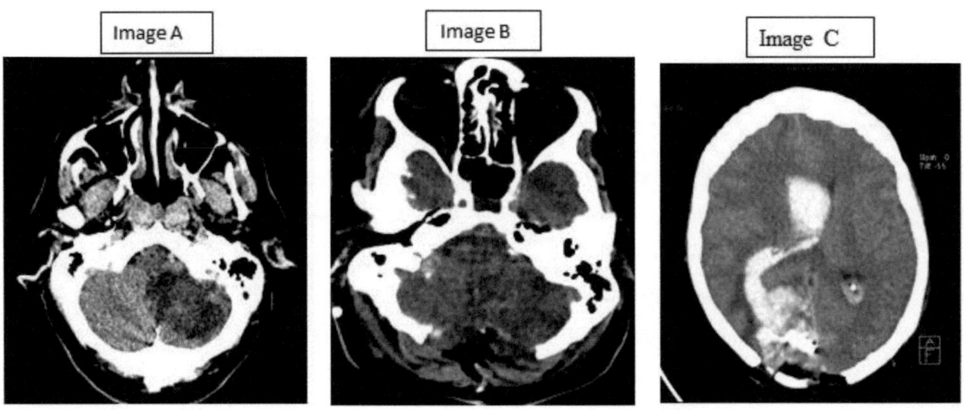

IMAGE "C" displayed is a cut of the cranial computed tomography of a 56-year-old woman with right occipital arteriovenous malformation. The patient during her stay in intensive care was complicated by acute myocardial infarction, cardiogenic shock, dying 12 days after her admission.

4. Results

Let us consider a moving window as shown in **Figure 2**.

For each moving windows, the correct value of τ and the embedding dimension N are calculated. Note that the last task means calculating the correlation integral for different dimensions of immersion, as shown in **Figure 2**.

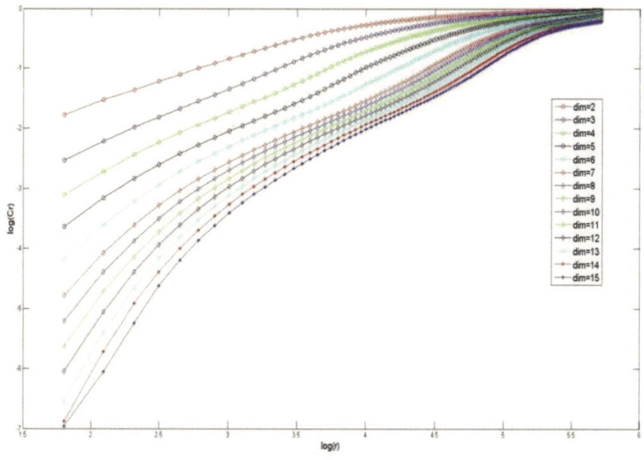

Figure 2. Correlation integrals for different embedding dimensions.

Once the appropriate dimension of embedding for each mobile window was calculated, we calculated the corresponding correlation dimension. In total, between sick and healthy people we amount 96,508 mobile windows of 5000 points each. We decided to choose the length of the mobile window equal to 5000 because we have observed that for that distance the average value of the mutual information function is practically zero, which indicates that over the time series, values separated by 5000 units of time or more have any correlation.

With these data, we calculate the probability density functions of the corresponding windows for healthy and sick behaviors. The results appear in **Figure 3**.

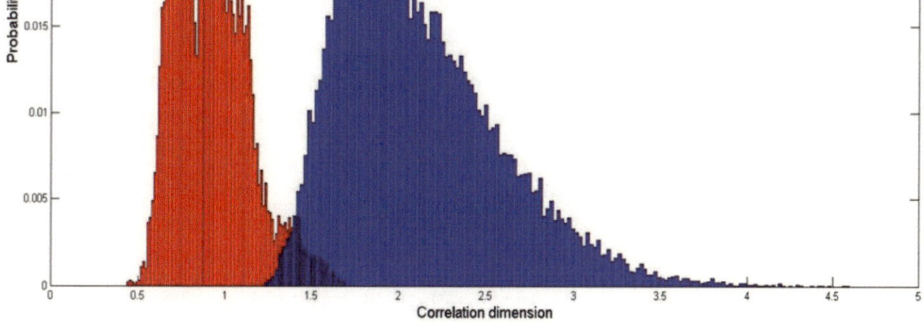

Figure 3. Probability density functions of correlation dimensions for windows sick (clearer) behavior an healthy (darker) behavior.

Note that there is a clear separation between the dimensions of correlation for sick and healthy behaviors. Finally, we note that small-dimensional correlation magnitudes are related to less complex behaviors than those with high correlation dimensions. It is important to note that in our database are records of people who were healthy and became in serious condition, as well as people who were sick and recovered later.

5. Discussion

The neural regulation of cardiac bioelectric signal has been explored in the frequency domain, showing the complexity of the sympathovagal balance which is tonically and phasically modulated by the interaction of at least three major factors: (a) central neural integration, (b) peripheral inhibitory reflex mechanisms (with negative-feedback characteristics), and (c) peripheral excitatory reflex mechanisms (with positive-feedback characteristics) [29]. Parasympathetic efferent nerve fibers come through the parasympathetic ganglia positioned in the periaortic and epicardial fat pad. Efferent sympathetic innervation arrives from superior, middle, and inferior cervical and the upper four or five thoracic ganglia. Medullary nuclei and reticular formation give both excitatory and inhibitory preganglionic efferent fibers as well as accept afferent fibers. Afferent pathways from baroreceptors and the so-called cardiopulmonary receptors to the brain stem are closing the loop assuring a feedback mechanism. These baroreceptors are located in the wall of aortic arch and great arteries arising from it, and in the carotid sinus. The hypothalamus is considered the most important supramedullary compound that integrates autonomic, somatic, mental, and emotional information via its extensive associations [29].

The applications of entropy on human physiological signals were developed earlier for analyzing the heart rate and beat-to-beat blood pressure. Heart rate is influenced by numerous factors including the liquid metabolism, hormonal and temperature variations, physical activity, circadian rhythms, and autonomic nervous system. As a result, heart rate variations are extremely complex in healthy individuals [37].

The entropy of heart rate was linked to neurological system since the modulation of heart beat was associated with the two components of autonomic nervous system: sympathetic and parasympathetic nerves [38]. Rhythmical oscillations of both heart rate and blood pressure have been indicated to reflect the sympathetic and parasympathetic modulation [39, 40].

The evaluation of the autonomic function provides important information about the alteration of the sympathetic-parasympathetic, altered balance in critically ill patients with or without multiple organ failure. The proven tools are heart rate variability, baroreflex sensitivity, and, with limitations, cardiac chemoreflex sensitivity [38]. The R-R interval functions as a substitute for the sympathovagal balance and represents the net result of all autonomic influences in the sinus node. Both the sympathetic and parasympathetic inputs to the sinus node can be characterized by a tonic level of activity and by the modulation of this activity (e.g., by respiration in the case of the parasympathetic input). Heart rate variability most reliably provides a measure of the modulation of the sympathetic and parasympathetic inputs to the sinus node, although a more precise way to characterize the sympathovagal balance is unknown [41, 42]. With new, nonlinear methods being evaluated, the risk (with prognostic implications) could be predicted more accurately by providing additional information on autonomic heart rate control in critically ill patients [29].

6. Conclusions

The results obtained allow us to arrive at the following conclusions: if the time windows studied belong to a person who is sick, the complexity of the time series is low, the dimension of embedding is small (below 6), and the dimension of correlation is low (below 2). For healthy people, the dimension of embedding is higher (above 7), the correlation dimension is also higher (above 2). The transition from a completely healthy to a completely sick behavior and vice versa occurs continuously. If the temporary moving windows corresponding to stages of transit between completely healthy and completely diseased behavior had been included in the analysis, such marked differences in the distributions of the correlation dimensions in each of these cases do not happen suddenly. In general, the heart electrical signal of a healthy person is more complex than that of a sick person. Results similar to these have been obtained by other methods [25]. In the aforementioned work, the authors affirm that the results obtained by them show that the cardiac dynamics of a healthy subject is more complex and random compared to the same for a heart failure patient, whose dynamics is more deterministic [43]. Our results are more general because we have managed to classify temporary windows in "healthy" or "diseased" (even for the same person) in terms of the complexity of the time series from their embedding dimension or their correlation dimension.

Our work opens the possibility of observing with these tools patients, for example, under anesthesia and relaxation in the operating room and critical care unit where patients often have no possibility of spoken communication, opening another way to evaluate and monitor the increase or decrease in the complexity of the cardiac bioelectrical signal, with the future possibility to evaluate the severity of the sick state or the reduction of this, analyzing in real time the behavior of the dynamics of that bioelectrical signal by means of the observation of the loss or recovery of the dimension of that bioelectrical signal, which is getting a numeric value that suggests the severity of the patient.

The implications of this for the early warning of the episodes of dysfunction are clear. Once the embedding dimension or the correlation dimension falls below a preset threshold, we may consider that we are facing an emergency.

Finally, the algorithms must deliver the results in real time in order for early warning to be effective and this is a challenge that must be faced. The ever-increasing speed of digital devices will certainly help this goal. On the other hand, the thresholds for early warnings should be obtained from careful statistical experiments.

Author details

Pedro Eduardo Alvarado Rubio[1], Ricardo Mansilla Corona[2], Lizette Segura Vimbela[1]*, Alejandro González Mora[1], Roberto Brugada Molina[3], Cesar Augusto González López[3] and Laura Yavarik Alvarado Avila[4]

*Address all correspondence to: merida_timucuy@yahoo.com.mx

1 Critical Care Unit Hospital Regional Lic., Adolfo López Mateos Social Security Institute for State Workers (ISSSTE), National Autonomous University of Mexico (UNAM), Mexico City, Mexico

2 Center for Interdisciplinary Research in the Sciences and Humanities (CEIICH), National Autonomous University of Mexico (UNAM), Mexico City, Mexico

3 Intensive Care Unit, Regional Hospital Lic, Adolfo López Mateos ISSSTE, Mexico City, Mexico

4 National Autonomous University of Mexico - Faculty of Veterinary Medicine, UNAM, Mexico City, Mexico

References

[1] Van der Pol B, Van der Mark J. Frequency demultiplication. Nature. 1927;**120**(3019):363-364

[2] Van der Pol B, van der Mark J. The heart beat considered as a relaxation oscillator, and an electrical model of the heart. Philosophical Magazine (Supplements). 1928;**6**:763-775

[3] Babloyantz A, Destexhe A. Is the normal heart a periodic oscillator? Journal of Biological Cybernetics. 1988;**58**:203-211

[4] Goldberger A, West B. Applications of nonlinear dynamics to clinical cardiology. Annals of New York Academy of Sciences. 1987;**504**:195-213

[5] Glass L, Mackey M. From Clock to Chaos: The Rhythms of Life. Princeton, NJ: Princeton University Press; 1988

[6] Guevara MR, Glass L, Shrier A. Phase locking, period-doubling bifurcations, and irregular dynamics in periodically stimulated cardiac cells. Science. 1981;**214**:1350-1353

[7] Garfinkel A. A mathematics for physiology. American Journal Physiology. 1983;**245**:R455-R466

[8] Ritzenberg A, Adam D, Cohen R. Period multiplying evidence for nonlinear behavior of the canine heart. Nature. 1984;**307**:159-161

[9] Small M, et al. Automatic identification and recording of cardiac arrhythmia. Computers in Cardiology. 2000;**27**:355-358

[10] Wolf M, Varigos G, Hunt D, Sloman J. Sinus arrhythmia in acute myocardial infarction. Medical Journal of Australia. 1978;**2**:52-53

[11] Kitney RI, Rompelman O. The Study of Heart Rate Variability. Oxford: Clarendon Press; 1980

[12] Kleiger RE, Miller JP, Bigger JT, Moss AR. Multicenter Post-infarction Research Group. Decreased heart rate variability and its association with increased mortality after acute myocardial infarction. American Journal of Cardiology. 1987;**59**:256-262

[13] Lombardi F, Porta A, Marzegalli M, Favale S, Santini M, Vincenti A, De Rosa A, and participating investigators of ICD-HRV Italian Study Group. Heart rate variability patterns before ventricular tachycardia onset in patients with an implantable cardioverter defibrillator. American Journal of Cardiology. 2000;**86**:959-963

[14] FitzHugh R. Impulses and physiological states in theoretical models of nerve membrane. Biophysical Journal. 1961;**1**:445-466

[15] Nagumo J, et al. An active pulse transmission line simulating nerve axon. Proceedings of IEEE. 1962;**50**:2061-2070

[16] Small M, et al. Automatic identification and recording of cardiac arrhythmia. Computers in Cardiology. 2000;**27**:355-358

[17] Venkatesh M, et al. Association of short term heart rate spectral power with onset of spontaneous ventricular tachycardia or ventricular fibrillation. Computers in Cardiology. 1998;**25**:101-104

[18] Ervin S, Lewis A. Necessity of noise in physiology and medicine. Computer Methods and Programs in Biomedicine. 2013;**111**:459-470

[19] Small M, et al. Deterministic nonlinearity in ventricular fibrillation. Chaos. 2000;**10**:268-277

[20] Zhang XSh, et al. Detecting ventricular tachycardia and fibrillation by complexity measure. IEEE Transactions on Biomedical Engineering. 1999;**46**:548-555

[21] Hon EH, Lee ST. Electronic evaluation of the fetal heart rate. VIII. Patterns preceding fetal death, further observations. American Journal of Obstetrics and Gynecology. 1963 Nov 15;**87**:814-826

[22] Kobayashi M, Musha T. 1/f fluctuation of heartbeat period. IEEE Transactions on Biomedical Engineering. 1982;**29**:456-457

[23] Goldberger A, Rigney D, Mietus J, Antman E, Greenwald S. Nonlinear dynamics in sudden cardiac death syndrome: Heart rate oscillations and bifurcations. Experientia. 1988;**44**:983-987

[24] Goldberger A. Is the normal heartbeat chaotic or homeostatic? News in Physiological Science. 1991;**6**:87-91

[25] Voss A, Schulz S, Schroeder R, Baumert M, Caminal P. Methods derived from nonlinear dynamics for analyzing heart rate variability. Philosophical Transactions of the Royal Society A. 2009;**367**:277-296

[26] Norris PR, Anderson SM, Jenkins JM, Williams AE, Morris Jr, JA. Heart rate multiscale entropy at three hours predicts hospital mortality in 3,154 trauma patients. Shock. 2008;**30**:17-22

[27] Bär K-J, Boettger MK, Koschke M, Schulz S, Chokka P, Yeragani VK, Voss A. Non-linear complexity measures of heart rate variability in acute schizophrenia. Clinical Neurophysiology. 2007;**118**:2009-2015

[28] Bar KJ, Letzsch A, Jochum T, Wagner G, Greiner W, Sauer H, et al. Loss of efferent vagal activity in acute schizophrenia. Journal of Psychiatric Research. 2005;**39**:519-527

[29] Hejjel L, Gál I. Heart rate variability analysis. Acta Physiologica Hungarica. 2001;**88**:219-230

[30] Amaral LAN, Goldberger AL, Ivanovc PCh, Stanley HE. Modeling heart rate variability by stochastic feedback. Computer Physics Communications. 1999;**121–122**:126-128

[31] Berne RM, Levy MN. Cardiovascular Physiology. 6th ed. St. Louis: C.V. Mosby; 1996

[32] Takens F. Detecting strange attractors in turbulence. In: Rand D, Young L, editors. Springer Lecture Notes in Mathematics. Vol. 898. 1981. pp. 366-381

[33] Small M. Applied Nonlinear Time Series Analysis. Applications in Physics, Physiology and Finance. World Scientific Publishing; 2005

[34] Shannon C. A mathematical theory of communication. The Bell System Technical Journal. 1948;**27**:3

[35] Fraser A, Swinney H. Independent coordinates for strange attractors from mutual information. Physical Review A. 1986;**33**(2):1134-1140

[36] Celluci C, et al. Statistical validation of mutual information calculations: Comparison of alternative numerical algorithms. Physical Review E. 2005;**71**:066208

[37] Kaplan DT, Furman MI, Pincus SM, Ryan SM, Lipsitz LA, Goldberger AL. Aging and the complexity of cardiovascular dynamics. Biophysical Journal. 1991;**59**(4):945-949

[38] Malliani A, Pagani M, Lombardi F, Cerutti S. Cardiovascular neural regulation explored in the frequency domain. Circulation. 1991;**84**(2):482-492

[39] Pagani M, Lombardi F, Guzzetti S, et al. Power spectral analysis of heart rate and arterial pressure variabilities as a marker of sympatho-vagal interaction in man and conscious dog. Circulation Research. 1986;**59**(2):178-193

[40] Malliani A, Montano N. Heart rate variability as a clinical tool. Italian Heart Journal. 2002;**3**(8):439-445

[41] Goldberger JJ. Sympathovagal balance: How should we measure it? American Journal of Physiology—Heart and Circulatory Physiology. 1 April 1999;**276**(4)

[42] Schmidt H, et al. Impaired chemoreflex sensitivity in adult patients with multiple organ dysfunction syndrome: The potential role of disease severity. Intensive Care Medicine. 2004;**30**:665-672

[43] Mukherlee S, et al. Can complexity decrease in congestive heart failure? Physica A. 2015;**439**:93-102